ESSENTIALS FOR MEN

sex & lifestyle

mike walsh

ESSENTIALS FOR MEN: SEX & LIFESTYLE

Mike Walsh

First published in 2000 by Mitchell Beazley,
an imprint of Octopus Publishing Group Ltd
2–4 Heron Quays, London EI4 4JP
Copyright © Octopus Publishing Group Ltd 2000

Executive Editor	Rachael Stock
	Vivien Antwi
Executive Art Editor	Kenny Grant
Project Editor	Jane Cooke
	Michelle Bernard
Art Editor	Christine Keilty
Design	Lovelock & Co
Production	Nancy Roberts
Picture Research	Jenny Faithfull
	Lois Charlton
Index	Hilary Bird
Illustrations	Jim Robbins
	Halli Verrinder
Special Photography	Steve Gorton
Medical Consultant	Dr Abi Berger, MRCGP

All rights reserved. No part of this work may be reproduced
or utilized in any form or by any means, electronic or mechanical,
including photocopying, recording or by any information
storage and retrieval system, without the prior written
permission of the publisher.

ISBN 1 84000-320-0

A CIP catalogue record for this book is available from
the British Library.

Front cover: Getty One Stone/Uwe Kreijci

Typeset in Flyer, Impact and Syntax

Printed in China
by Toppan Printing Company Ltd

ESSENTIALS FOR MEN

sex & lifestyle

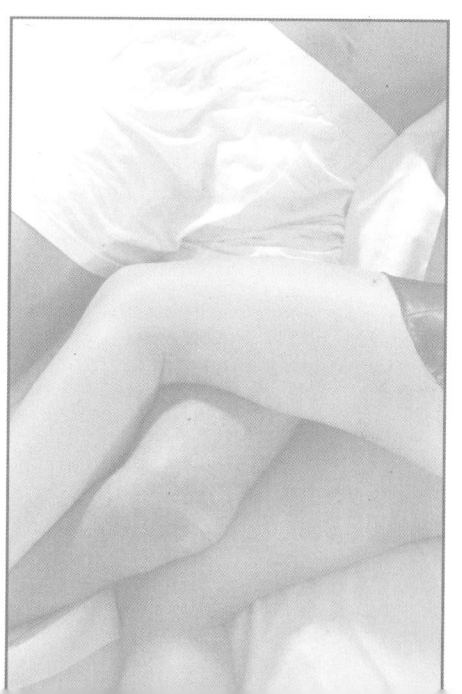

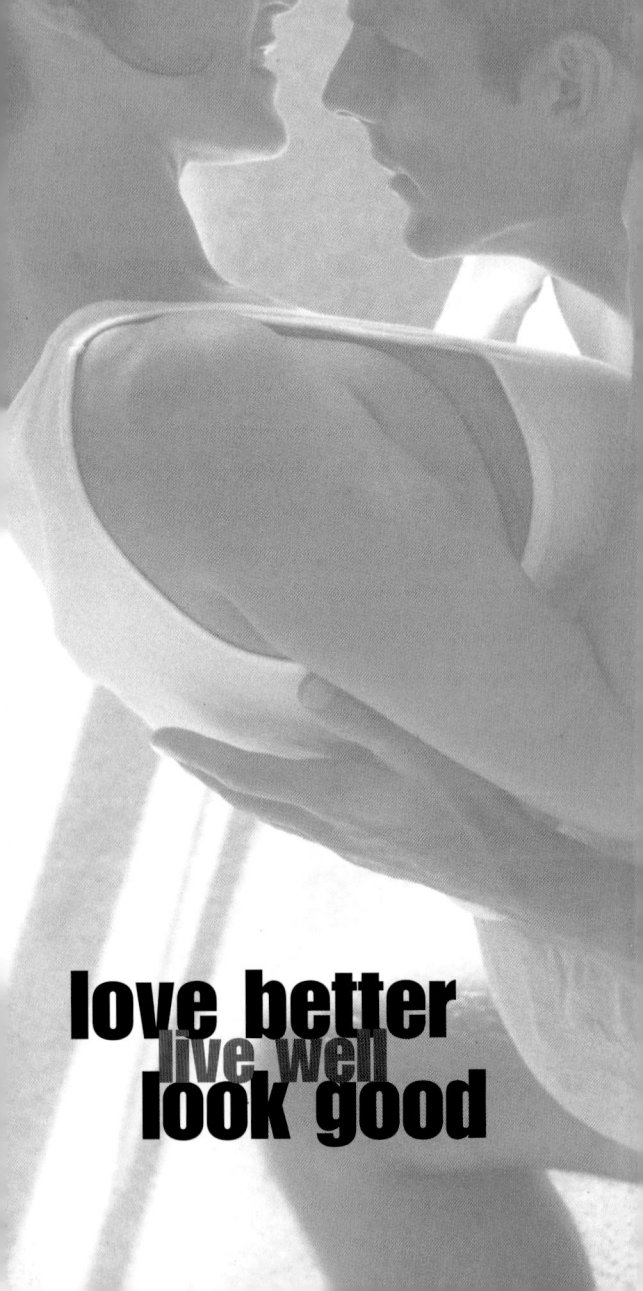

Contents

Introduction

Life matters

12 Changing your life
14 Taking control
16 Getting out of a rut
18 Breaking bad habits
20 Slowing down ageing
22 Sleeping easy
24 Are you stressed?
26 Reducing stress
28 Are you a workaholic?
30 Managing work
32 Learning to relax

Looking good

36 Smooth and sexy skin
40 Healthy hair
42 Stylish hair
44 Dealing with hair loss
46 Hair elsewhere
50 Smelling fresh
52 Oral hygiene
56 Male nails

The right diet

60 Eating for life
62 Major food groups
64 Vital vitamins
66 Must-have minerals
68 The food pyramid
70 Planning what you eat
72 Weighty matters
74 Shedding the flab
76 Drinking to your health
78 Organic eating
80 Food supplements

Nurturing relationships

84 Communicating well
86 Body language
88 The art of listening
90 Understand one another
92 Revisiting passion
94 Keeping love alive
96 Back in the market

First impressions

100 First moves
102 Dressing with sense
104 Suits you sir
106 First base to home run

Great sex

110 Puberty
112 Masturbation
114 Losing it
116 Sexual psychology
118 Foreplay
122 Massage
124 Sensual massage
126 Oral sex
130 Sexual phases
132 Male orgasms
134 Female orgasms
136 Moving the earth
138 Multiple orgasms
140 Alternatives to intercourse
142 Games and fantasies
146 Sexual aids
148 Dressing for sex
150 Potency
152 Aphrodisiacs
154 Dealing with impotency
156 Contraceptive methods
164 Sexual health

Sex manual

170 Creative lovemaking
172 Missionary variations
174 Basic positions
176 Face-to-face positions
178 Rear-entry positions
180 Advanced positions
182 Athletic positions

184 Index
192 Acknowledgements

Introduction

This book has a simple aim: to help you improve your life and enjoy better sex. Many of us today live such a frenetic lifestyle that we fail to notice how being busy isn't necessarily the same as being happy. Pressures at work and the demands of parents, wives, girlfriends, and children can cause stress and compromise our emotional well being.

This book offers no panacea to these problems. Nor does it provide definitive medical advice – for any health problem, however large or small, you are strongly advised to consult your doctor. But it does give guidance on how to reduce stress, improve relationships, and have an even better time in bed.

About this book

The book is divided into six main chapters. The first five cover lifestyle issues such as work and relaxation, looking after yourself physically, food and diet, and starting and maintaining relationships. The last chapter covers just about everything to do with sex, from puberty and masturbation to foreplay, massage, sex games, contraception and sexual health. Finally, the section on sex positions should spark ideas for both the laziest and most athletic of men.

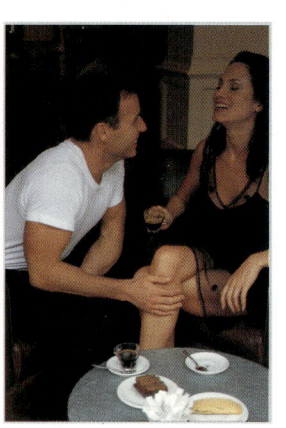

Changing your life

Do you control your life or does your life control you? The key commitments of most people's lives are at home and at work. There was once a time when you made the choices. Now, work and home may have gained a momentum of their own. Your wife or girlfriend wants to spend more time with you, while your boss gives you ever more work. All of which results in stress.

Stress

The chapter on changing your life will show you how to deal with stress. It may well be that you need to look up from your desk for long enough to reassess your life. Is your partner becoming something of a stranger because you are getting home ever later from work? Are you forgetting friends' birthdays? Are you smoking or drinking more? Things can change – and may have to if you want to avoid long-term medical and emotional problems. You just need to be determined to get out of the rut. That may even mean considering changing jobs. Such a step could seem radical but consider this: no one on their death bed has ever said they wished they'd spent more time at work.

Looking good

Even the least vain man feels good about himself when he knows he's looking fit and healthy. In recent years men have come under increasing pressure to look after themselves better. The range of health care products has proliferated. Cosmetics manufacturers have created a multitude of new and better products, hair gels, deodorants and a host of other items. Some are useful, some are just plain exploitative. More important is how you take care of yourself. The second chapter gives tips on how to look after your skin and hair. It also suggests the type of haircut that should best suit your shape of face. There are tips on trimming beards and keeping your breath fresh. There is also advice on how to get the best shave, how to look after your teeth, and even how to cut your nails. Put all these tips into practice and before you know it you'll be turning heads in the street.

The right diet

Your mum was right: finishing your greens and not scoffing too many chips was sound advice. But many of us still pay too little attention to what we eat. The body's extraordinary resilience can mask the damage you may be causing it. But in the long run, failure to consume the right nutrients will surely take its toll.

Food contains the raw materials necessary to repair the body and also provides the fuel for energy. The key elements you need are carbohydrates, protein, fat, vitamins, minerals, fibre, and water. You do not need to learn exactly which nutrients are provided by every type of food. But having a broad understanding of what food types will supply the carbohydrates, protein, vitamins, and minerals you require will make it easier to ensure you maintain a balanced diet and get what you need.

Knowing how much to eat is also important. There's advice on how to lose weight and how to keep a check on your alcoholic intake. The aim is not to spoil your enjoyment of food but to build up an appetite for the healthier options that not only taste good but also stay off your waist.

Relationships

A warm and loving relationship with your partner is probably the most emotionally fulfilling experience you can have. But attaining it can be something of a holy grail. At school you learned all about algebra and the periodic table but nothing about how to communicate properly with the opposite sex or how to nurture a relationship. For many teenagers – and indeed men – making the first move can be a huge hurdle. Our book makes this less of a guessing game and gives practical, down-to-earth tips.

Communication

Take a look at the list of where to meet single women and where to go on a date. Observing a potential partner's body language, and keeping a check on your own, is also a useful skill. And what about once you are in a relationship? The throes of passion and desire can propel you through the early days but how well do you really communicate? Women and men are notorious for failing to understand each other properly. But by learning how your partner tends to react and understanding her fundamental concerns, you can avoid conflict and build a relationship based on love and trust.

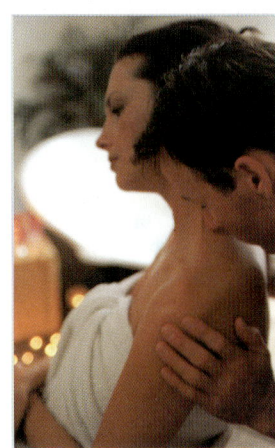

Great sex

Sex is a wonderful and life-affirming experience when done in the right place at the right time. Many men might also say it's pretty good when done in the wrong place at the wrong time. Joking aside, you can never know too much about sex.

For a subject that is a favourite preoccupation of the male mind, it is remarkable how ignorant many men are of their own sexual response and their partner's, contraception, and sexual health. Many might also be chastened to hear how unimaginative their partners say they are between the sheets.

Tips

The chapter on great sex moves through the bedroom door to show you how to improve your foreplay techniques, how to give a good massage, and how to give good oral sex. It also offers tips on strengthening orgasm, delaying ejaculation, and dealing with impotence. For would-be actors there is a list of suggested role-playing scenarios, plus a look at the merits of claimed aphrodisiacs.

But sex of course is not without its responsibilities. Unless you and your partner wish to have a baby, make sure you always use some form of contraception and always practise safe sex. Life is to be lived. So look after yourself – and those around you – and go and live it.

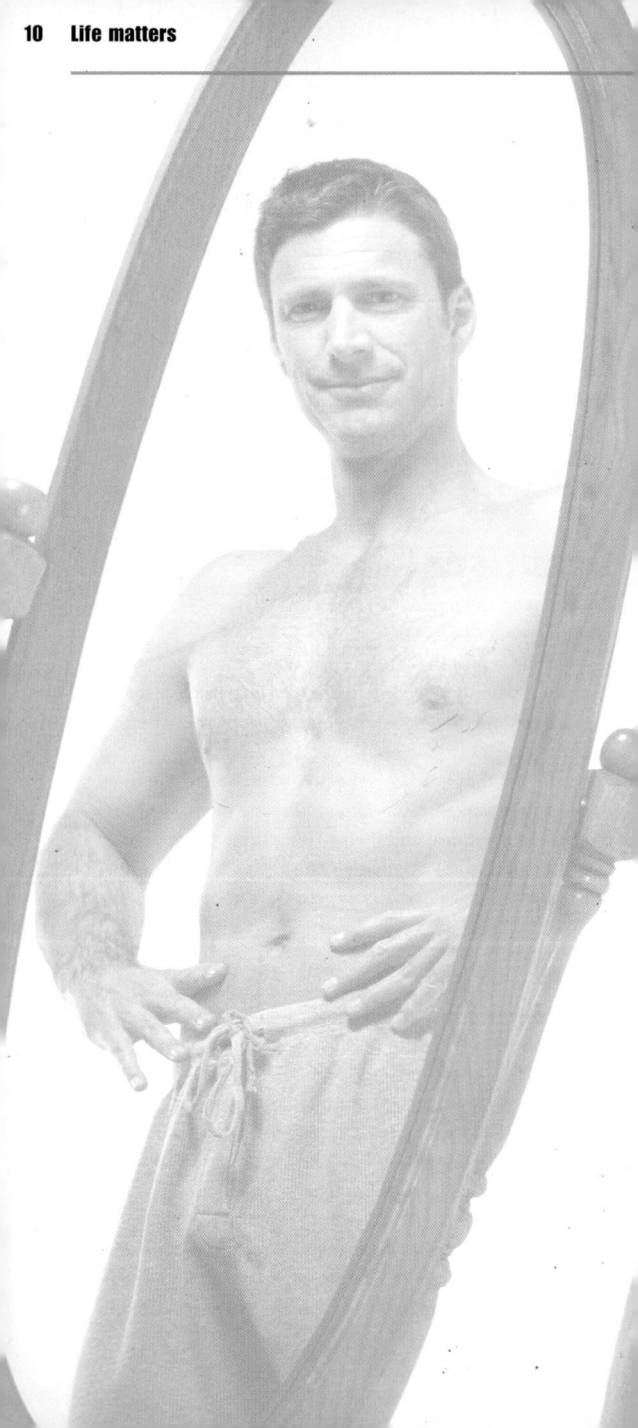

Life matters

Changing your life
Taking control
Getting out of a rut
Breaking bad habits
Slowing down ageing
Sleeping easy
Are you stressed?
Reducing stress
Are you a workaholic?
Managing work
Learning to relax

Changing your life

Looking after a marriage, children, mortgage, and career can take a lot of juggling. But step back and assess your values. You may find your life need not be such a circus.

Time to take stock

- The high pace of modern life can leave you with little time to assess what really matters. You may think friends and family are top of your list, but analyse how often you see them. If pressure at work makes you forget an important birthday, it may be time to re-examine your values.
- The desire to be in control of your career by striving for promotion may leave you lacking control of your personal life. Such an unbalanced life can lead to a host of problems and impede the very progress at work that you strive for.

Love or money?

- Most of us want love and money. But the pursuit of the latter can bring out aggressive characteristics that should be left behind in the office and not taken home with you.
- Recognise that working late and refusing to take holidays are forms of workaholism. Try to resist them. Reduce your work load, make more time for yourself, and find more time for your wife and family. Let them connect with you without making them feel they're imposing on you. You'll be much the richer for it.

Marriage facts

Marriage is good for your health – it's official. One research study found that the mortality rate among unmarried men in the Western world was about twice as high as that among married men. Married men were also found to have fewer mental and physical illnesses and were generally happier.

Do you want to change?

Choosing to live a better, healthier life is likely to require a fresh mental approach. You'll need to identify your priorities and pay attention to your emotions. How you spend your time is a yardstick of what you value. If you answer yes to five or more of the following questions, you may want to consider changing your lifestyle.

1. Do you think others find you boring?

2. Do you use a holiday as a time to catch up on work and domestic chores?

3. Can you tell if that nagging empty feeling in your stomach is hunger or anxiety? Do you know if you are sweating from the heat or from panic?

4. Do you mainly eat things you can hold in your hand while writing, walking along the street, talking on the 'phone, or driving? Are you overindulging in junk or processed food, cigarettes, or alcohol?

5. Do you often turn down invitations to social events because you can't face them?

6. Do you feel anxious if work is delegated to anyone else?

7. Are you ignoring aches and pains that probably ought to be investigated and treated?

8. Does anxiously looking at your watch dictate where you'll be all day long?

9. Do you often volunteer to do extra tasks at work and stay late rather than go home and face what you'll find there? Do you have trouble remembering when you last saw your neighbourhood in daylight?

10. Do you feel as though there is always something missing in your life?

Taking control

Do you run your life or does your life run you? Regaining control can be a challenge, but the merits of a balanced physical and emotional life are worth pursuing.

Know your body

Just as your car splutters and chokes when something's wrong, so your body sends out distress signals. Ignoring them is likely to lead to trouble. If you feel pain for prolonged periods or develop unfamiliar lumps, sores, or aches that don't disappear within a few days, see a doctor.

Meet your doctor

With prevention being preferable to cure, you should overcome the male reluctance to visit the doctor. There is no merit in stoically enduring an illness. A good doctor will explain the cause of your illness and how to treat it.

Recognise your emotions

- Men who define themselves by their work often do so by losing touch with their emotional side. Many men at work learn to keep their emotions in check while striving for power and promotion.
- Today's corporate environment of takeovers and downsizing sharpens your survival instincts at the expense of the caring characteristics that your friends and family value.
- Many men choose punishing careers because the pay may be better – but most wives and family would rather see more of you than more money.
- Failure to balance work with family life and pleasure time can lead to a wide range of problems, including the inability to develop the social skills that are probably essential in achieving the career stature you crave.

Top ten tips for total health

Here are ten key areas you should focus on for a healthier, happier, and more balanced lifestyle:

1. **Don't smoke** It's not good for your lungs or heart – or for anybody else's.

2. **Eat well** Reduce your calorie intake and limit the amount of fat, sugar, and salt in your diet. Eat plenty of fibre and fruit and vegetables with more complex carbohydrates, such as potatoes, pasta, rice, and bread.

3. **Be moderate** Practise moderation, especially with alcohol consumption – binge drinking is particularly damaging.

4. **Exercise regularly** And stick at it. Vary your activities as this will exercise different sets of muscles and reduce the monotony of just one type of workout.

5. **Maintain a healthy weight** Being overweight aggravates high blood pressure and heart disease. You are also more likely to sweat profusely, particularly in warm weather.

6. **Exercise your mind** Have a good conversation with a friend or learn something new. Connect with some power greater than yourself – be it God or the great outdoors.

7. **Be positive** Have a good mental attitude. Learn to laugh at petty annoyances. Keep problems in perspective and save your real angst for serious upsets.

8. **Monitor your health** See your doctor about any worrying symptoms and carry out self-examinations monthly.

9. **Look after your teeth** Brush them regularly, including the roof of your mouth and your tongue. Keep a toothbrush at work, and remember to floss regularly to loosen those difficult-to-reach bits of food.

10. **Get plenty of sleep** Experts say men need 8–9 hours a night. Get into the habit of going to bed at the same time.

Getting out of a rut

It's very easy to get into a routine of working long hours and going home to guzzle something unhealthy in front of the TV. But you can choose to live your life differently.

Ten ways to get out

1. **Think big** Try to delegate low-level jobs to others and leave them alone to get on without interfering. Delegating will both reduce your workload and empower you.

2. **Say no** Learn to say no to unreasonable demands. Set sensible limits for yourself and stick to them.

3. **Be easy on yourself** Know the difference between the demands of the job and the demands you make on yourself.

4. **Assess work** If tasks are added to your workload that will overwhelm you, speak to your boss sooner rather than later.

5. **Set realistic goals** Establish them for work and home.

6. **Get a life** Make a conscious effort to spend more time with family members and friends.

7. **Go out and play** Walk, run, swim, cycle, skate – even dig out that old train set from your childhood – whatever makes you relax. Playing will help to relieve stress, strengthen your heart and body, and give you a sense of well-being.

8. **Choose life** Give up smoking, cut down on drinking, eat a variety of food, keep your weight down, and laugh a lot!

9. **Find the right job** It's far less stressful to work at something you enjoy and that you're good at.

10. **Don't wait to enjoy life** Make time now – unless you're utterly fulfiled by your work, don't let it obscure the important things in life, like strong, close relationships.

Positive mental attitude

- It's all in the mind. If you think you can't do something, chances are you won't be able to do it. If you think you might be able to, you probably will. Getting out of a rut can take a lot of will-power and what feels like a long time.
- The key is to recognise that change always takes time. Like going on a diet it won't happen overnight, so don't expect it to. Set yourself a series of realistic targets and tackle them one by one. As you clear each hurdle, the finish line will get nearer. With a positive view you can be on well on track to change tack.

Top tips for staying out

1. **Set limits** And stick to them. If you've decided to spend more time with your family, remind yourself of that priority. Visualise how happy your wife and kids are to see you get home when you say you will, and how disappointed they'll be if you call again to say you're running late. Once at home, don't spoil things by polluting the atmosphere with your stress from work.

2. **Limit work hours** Decide how many hours a week you want to work and then stop when you've reached that limit. This may not always be possible but try to tailor your job so that it is regularly achievable. If you're working as efficiently as possible – that is not wasting time gossiping and surfing the internet – but still struggling to limit your working hours, consult your manager or superior.

3. **Who's boss?** If you start to feel your life spinning out of control, remind yourself that you're driving your life, rather than your boss. If your workload requires 60–70 hours a week as standard, consider changing job or career.

4. **Positive change** Remind yourself that the right kind of change that you control and that's aimed at improving your quality of life, can be invigorating rather than stressful.

5. **Pass it up** Consider passing up the next promotion opportunity, especially if means more working hours.

Breaking bad habits

Many of us resort to a range of unhealthy habits to cope with the stresses of everyday life. But living a healthy life means giving up such habits. It can take time, but it's worth it.

Smoke in your eyes

- If you smoke you'll know this – you shouldn't. Give up now. It's the fastest, sure-fire way to improve your health.
- Cigarettes and cigars contain at least 40 carcinogenic chemicals and they reduce the amount of oxygen the lungs can carry to the blood.
- Still not convinced? Smoking makes you 22 times more likely to die from lung cancer.

Aids to quitting

- Commit yourself. Decide that smoking is not an option.
- You can try steadily cutting down but this doesn't always work. Many doctors believe the best way to beat the weed is to stop altogether.
- Throw out all objects associated with smoking, such as ashtrays and lighters at home, work, and in the car.
- Get a friend to quit at the same time as you or join a local support group.
- Consider a nicotine skin patch. These can help you adjust to life without cigarettes.

Care with caffeine

- Many of us rely on a cup of coffee to kick-start us in the morning. Caffeine, the magic ingredient, is a mild stimulant that can improve mental alertness, concentration, and memory.
- There are, however, downsides. The best advice is to cut back if your coffee intake makes you nervous or irritable, or if it disturbs your sleep.

The demon drink

- Moderation, as with most enjoyable things in life, is what's required when it comes to boozing. A bit of alcohol can be good for you. But guzzling more than three glasses of beer or wine a day can harm your health, as well as your professional and personal well being.
- Try to meet friends in a café or at the cinema instead of always in a pub to help you stick to drinking within safe limits.

Sex 'n' booze: the benefits

Choosing sexual partners carefully and monitoring your alcohol intake mean sex and booze can be good for you!

SEX
Intercourse can relieve stress, relax your body, help you sleep, stimulate your nervous system, boost your immune system, and keep you on an emotional even keel. But be careful if you're changing your partners. In this age of Aids and other sexually-transmitted diseases, one night of passion can haunt you forever. Always use a condom, and remember, some people may be unaware that they are carriers of the HIV virus.

BOOZE
Alcohol is only good for you if you keep your drinking under control. Studies show that moderate drinkers have healthier hearts and live longer than heavy drinkers or abstainers. Alcohol can protect you against heart disease. It increases the level of HDL cholesterol, which helps carry away the artery clogging "bad" LDL cholesterol. It's also been found that alcohol decreases the blood's ability to form clots, which block blood vessels and cause heart attacks and strokes. The key, as ever, is moderate consumption. You should have no more than three units of alcohol a day. That's one-and-a-half pints of beer, three glasses of wine, or three pub measures of spirits. Keep your drinking within safe limits and stick to them.

Slowing down ageing

However much you fight it, as you age your body starts to wear out. And from your late twenties your metabolic rate slows down, which means you start putting on the pounds.

The ageing process

- Your skin, which once quickly replaced itself, now hangs around for longer. Your hair begins to lose its colour as the body's supply of pigment decreases and, less visibly, many of your vital organs are in decline as cells in the kidneys, brain, heart, and eyes stop renewing themselves.
- Bones and muscles gradually weaken due to reduced levels of elastin and possibly also testosterone.

Diet and exercise

- You can't halt the ageing process, but you can put the brakes on it. A slower metabolism means you should reduce your calorie intake to head off an expanding waistline.
- Eat fewer fatty foods and protein, such as red meat, but more grains, fruit, and vegetables, and combine this with three to five 30-minute aerobic sessions a week, such as swimming or cycling.

How to look and feel young

- Give up smoking.
- Avoid binge-drinking.
- Eat a moderate, low-fat diet.
- Exercise regularly – try going to the gym or running in your lunch hour.
- Protect yourself from the sun with sun screen. Sunlight is the skin's worst enemy.
- Reduce stress levels because stress damages heart and muscle tissue.
- Stay mentally active.

Free radicals

- What are free radicals? They are essentially on a mission to damage you. Molecular by-products of breathing, they are unstable, highly reactive, and they need electrons to survive. They gain electrons from your body tissue, leaving damaged cells behind. Those damaged cells lead to the diseases of ageing, such as cataracts, clogged arteries, and cancer.
- Fight back with antioxidants. Free radicals can be countered by antioxidants, as there is some evidence to suggest that antioxidants combat the tissue oxidation that free radicals cause. The principal antioxidants are vitamins C and E; beta-carotene, which the body turns into vitamin A; and the mineral selenium, which works in tandem with vitamin E. Others include vitamin B6, thiamin, lecithin, and zinc.

There is a view, which is unsubstantiated by medical research, that when taken in doses slightly higher than the recommended daily allowance, these nutrients help slow down the ageing process.

- Antioxidants are found mainly in fruit, vegetables, and whole grains. Natural sources include fresh vegetables, oats, wheat, rice and corn, garlic and onions, liver, kidney, fish, shellfish, red meat and poultry, citrus fruits, and berries.

Stay sharp

- Don't become a crotchety old man before your time. Leave that cynical outlook on life to the Victor Meldrews of this world.
- Stay mentally sharp by keeping up to date with current affairs and other mentally absorbing interests. Tackle those hard crosswords, learn a foreign language, or do some research on the internet. You could set aside time to travel more often and further afield.
- Although you will lose brain cells as you get older, a slowdown in memory recall will be offset by a satisfying rise in wisdom. Above all, make a constant effort to keep up with change and try to interact with people who are more intelligent than you.

Sleeping easy

Sleeping can seem such a waste of time. If only we didn't have to switch off, we could do so much more in life. Scientists still aren't sure why we need to sleep. But to operate at your mental and physical best, you know you need those sweet dreams.

Why you need sleep

- Without enough sleep, human performance decreases. That much is obvious to most of us. When you stay up past midnight to work on a report, you know how your vision gets blurred, your eyelids become heavy, and your brain seems to adopt the texture of soup. Your body is telling you to shutdown.
- Your mental agility becomes seriously affected with fatigue – your mood, performance, creativity, and ability to think critically all suffer.
- Under extreme conditions, no amount of willpower can keep humans awake. Dependency on an alarm clock is another symptom of sleep deprivation. If you need an alarm to rouse you every morning, then you're simply not getting enough shut-eye. Wake up to the fact that you need more sleep.

How much do you need?

- You probably need more sleep than you're getting. The average man sleeps for about seven hours a night – but he really needs eight to nine in order to stay fully alert.
- When you try to get by with less than eight to nine hours sleep, you miss out on the most important sleep cycle – the one that occurs between the seventh and eighth hours of sleep. During that time the brain's neural (nerve) network is stimulated, which is the equivalent of recharging the brain's batteries. This allows you to retain and regain new insights and it strengthens your memory.
- Missing out on sleep stops you performing at your peak because you miss out on the neural stimulation needed for memory and problem-solving.

Top ten tips for better sleep

1. **Be regular** Go to bed and get up at the same time every day, regardless of whether you have to go to work.

2. **Abstain** Avoid alcohol and cigarettes for at least 2 hours and coffee for 5 hours before going to bed.

3. **Bedroom sanctuary** Make your bedroom cosy and restful. Don't eat, work, or watch TV in it. Decorate it using warm, relaxing colours that are not too vibrant. At night your room should be as dark as possible. Make sure your curtains block out street lighting adequately.

4. **Move around** If you're having trouble falling asleep, don't just toss and turn. Get out of bed or go into another room. Read the small print on your house insurance form or, better still, do a few stretches. These will gently tire you out while relaxing the muscles at the same time.

5. **Avoid drugs** Try to avoid sleep-inducing drugs – they can become a bad habit, which you may have trouble breaking.

6. **Avoid food** Don't eat a heavy meal before you go to bed.

7. **Keep active** Exercise will help tire you out, making it easier to get to sleep. But for your body to recover, you should finish exercising at least 3 hours before bedtime.

8. **Close the day** Play some relaxing music, let some fresh air into the room, turn off the 'phone, and allow your body and mind to wind down for at least 30 minutes before you want to fall asleep. Some people find writing a diary is a good way of "closing" the day.

9. **Cat nap** If possible, take a 30-minute nap during the day when you're feeling tired.

10. **Limit your work** Don't rob yourself of rest by working late. When you've reached the limit of your productivity, call it a night. And be sure to mentally leave your work behind when you go home.

Are you stressed?

Grumpy bosses, late trains, and stroppy friends can make you feel stressed, propelling you on a downward spiral of pressure. Help is at hand but first you need to understand stress.

Warning signs

Ignore these stress signals and your health could suffer:
- Difficulty falling asleep
- Inability to concentrate, or lapses of concentration
- Reduced interest in sex
- Eating when not hungry, or not feeling hungry
- Smoking more
- Drinking more alcohol
- Recurrent headaches
- Increasing irritability, impatience, and loss of temper
- Constantly feeling lethargic

Is stress making you ill?

Heart disease Anxiety can cause your blood vessels to constrict and your heart rate to increase, eventually leading to high blood pressure and heart disease.

Digestive disorders Stress is known to contribute to gastrointestinal problems, such as chronic heart burn and irritable bowel syndrome.

Aches and pains Stress can aggravate back pain, and prolonged tension in the neck and shoulders can lead to headaches. This can be aggravated by incorrect posture.

Skin disorders In some people, stress causes skin rashes. Sitting in front of a radiation-emitting computer screen for long hours can also generate skin complaints, particularly on the cheeks and around the eyes.

Take the stress test

Your life ought to be a product of the choices you make. Are you choosing stress and anxiety or are you opting to feel relaxed and in control? Try the stress test below. If you answer yes to most of the positive choices questions, you're doing well. If not, it may be time to consider making some important changes in your life.

NEGATIVE CHOICES
- Do you get nervous, angry, or upset over small problems?
- Do you suffer from recurring headaches?
- Do your back and neck muscles ache constantly?
- Do you chain-smoke your way through the day?
- Are you overworked, lonely, or isolated?
- Do you regularly suffer from sleeping problems, shallow breathing, digestive problems, or high blood pressure?
- Do you constantly find fault with other people?
- Are you difficult to get along with or work with?
- Is your anger often out of proportion to the problem?
- Do you find it impossible to admit mistakes or to apologise to others?
- Do you become obsessed about wrongs you feel others have done to you? Do you feel victimised?

POSITIVE CHOICES
- Are you confident that you're giving your best efforts, and that your best is good enough?
- Do you have reasonable life objectives and goals?
- Do you ask for help readily?
- Do you walk away from your desk every so often for reasons other than to go to the toilet or for a drink?
- Do you kiss your wife, hug your kids, and stroke your pet when you get home?
- Do you make time for your family?
- Do you have hobbies, read books, or listen to music?
- Do you regularly have a good laugh?
- Do you leave your job at the door when you get home?
- Do you take time in the day to eat, relax, and exercise?

Reducing stress

Identifying the cause of stress may be easy but it's how you deal with it that matters. The right attitude and a proactive response can help.

Understanding stress

Stress stems from experiences that cause upset, anger, or frustration. Everyone has pressure in their life, ranging from difficult bosses to screaming babies, which makes them feel stressed. If your enjoyment of life is hampered by stress, your body may be warning you that you're under too much pressure.

Stress – it's up to you

Stress does actually serve a purpose. A heavy workload may either force you to become more organised, or it may prompt you to look for a new job. In the same way, anxiety about the prospect of a serious illness might spur you to see a doctor regularly. Stress shows how life can be like a poker game – you may be dealt a bad hand but how you play it is up to you.

Fight or flight

When you're stressed your pulse and blood pressure increase as your body prepares for action. This chart shows varying stress levels during a typical working day.

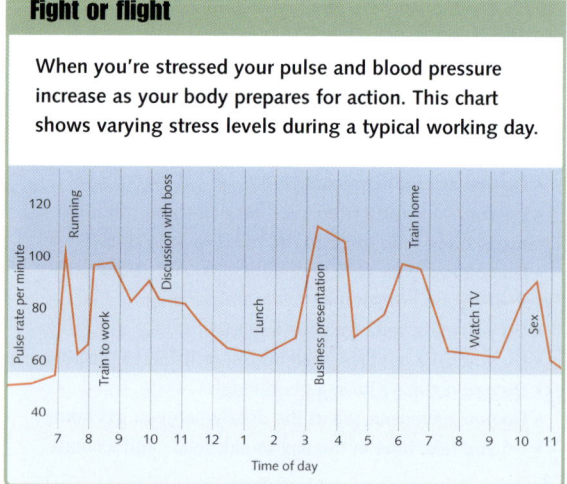

Stress busters: exercise, sleep, and good food

- **Exercise** Regular exercise not only keeps you fit but rids the body of stress-related hormones. Try to play a sport or activity for 30 minutes at least three times a week. If running becomes boring, mix it up with swimming, cycling, tennis, golf, brisk walking, or gardening.
- **Sleep** This is a tremendous antidote to stress, but is vastly under-rated by most men. Even napping for 30 minutes will refresh you, make you more alert, and get you started again.
- **Diet** Complex carbohydrates, such as rice, pasta, potatoes, and bread, generate serotonin in the brain, which helps to relieve stress, and give the body a steady source of energy. By eating a balanced diet, which also includes protein foods, fruit, and vegetables, your body will get all the nutrients it needs.

Top tips for a stress-free life

1 **Give yourself a break** Take time out for family, fun, and relaxation. All work and no play makes Jack a coronary risk.

2 **Quit smoking** Also reduce caffeine and alcohol intake.

3 **Chill out** Not every fight is worth winning. Stand your ground when you're right, but learn to give in graciously.

4 **Talk things out** If you're worried or under pressure, share it with a close friend, family member, or professional counsellor.

5 **Be reasonable** Assess what you can accomplish in a set time.

6 **Don't overspend** Watch your spending and live within your means, rather than using credit and living off expensive loans.

7 **Cry if you need to** Gazza's tears made crying fashionable again, although you may want a little more privacy for yours.

8 **Help someone out** It will take your mind off your troubles.

Are you a workaholic?

Do you regard work as a means to an end or as an end in itself? If work has taken over your life, you may have crossed that line. You have to ask yourself if it's worth it.

Self-assessment

Self-confessed workaholics speak of using work as a way of coping with life, just as alcoholics use alcohol. You could be a workaholic if:

- You work late nights, weekends, and you often take work home with you.
- You take work to bed with you.
- You feel guilty when you're not working.
- You refuse to take holidays.
- Your list of priorities fails to include family, friends, hobbies, and relaxation.
- You've started to forget important family occasions, such as birthdays and anniversaries.
- You have few friends, and not much social life outside your work circle.
- You live mainly on junk food.
- Your job gives you headaches and backaches, and your eyes are often sore.
- You're always accessible by employers or colleagues by mobile 'phone, pager, or email.
- It bothers you if you have to ask for help, no matter how complicated or difficult the task.
- You think a job won't be done properly unless you do it.
- You work to escape problems at home or in your personal life.
- Your own self-imposed expectations are your greatest source of pressure.
- You keep on accepting more work even when you're already over-committed.
- Work is your drug of choice.

The corporate jungle

- In today's corporate environment of hostile takeovers, downsizing, and outsourcing many of us have learned that survival has little to do with exhibiting the caring characteristics that are valued by our family and friends. It may seem paradoxical, but the office is not an environment in which most men feel in control.
- At work, most men learn to keep their emotions in check, while striving for power, promotion, kudos, and money. Some worry more about making themselves look good to their bosses rather than actually doing a good job. In such situations, men tend to shut down their emotional side and become harder and tougher.
- Hardened and toughened personalities can have terrible impacts on relationships. If production is the only thing you value, then you'll probably achieve high levels. But how productive are you if you jeopardise what should be more important – your relationships with those you love?

What's the point?

Striking a balance between work and your personal life can be difficult to achieve. But identifying your most important values can bring you closer to finding a solution. Consider the following questions:

- What do you want out of life?
- Do you define yourself by your job?
- Do you work long hours because you have to or because you are avoiding problems in your personal life?
- Do expensive cars and hotels matter to you?
- Do you value the time you spend at home with your partner and children?
- Do you feel that fulfilment at work is a poor substitute for a fulfilled private life?
- Does work give you a high that you can't get from relationships or other activities outside work?

If there's a big disparity between your priorities and how you actually spend your time, you may need to make changes in your life, including your career.

Managing work

Work can rule your life unless you make a conscious effort to manage it. Identify the tasks that really need doing and concentrate on them, leaving less important tasks to others or for another day when you're refreshed. Cut down on the office chat and the excess emails, and you should be well on your way to keeping work in perspective.

Eliminate the time-wasters

As well as finding ways to prevent stress, you can gain more control over your life with better time management. Sometimes the sheer volume of tasks to be done can seem overwhelming. The skill is to prioritise what really needs doing from the rest of the clutter. You should also find time for yourself. Reduce the amount of time you watch TV and do more creative activities that help to nourish your mind. When at work, try to tackle jobs one at a time without being side-tracked, and avoid recurring distractions that waste time.

You can be more productive at work by trying to avoid:
- Interruptions, especially 'phone calls
- Indecision
- Not having a plan for the day
- Gossiping too much
- Giving in to unreasonable demands
- Switching between tasks without completing them
- Meetings that take too long, particularly when much of what's being discussed doesn't affect you
- Poor communications – it's better to spend a little extra time spelling out what's required on a particular job clearly rather than assuming people know what you're talking about
- Minimising personal emails during working hours

Be realistic about work

- An excessive workload not only wears you out but it also has an impact on you emotionally as well as physically.
- Many men choose punishing careers because of some immature notion they have about male toughness.
- It's a modern truism that the work absenteeism of yesterday has been replaced by so-called presenteeism today.
- Men in the UK work considerably more hours per week on average than their European counterparts.
- The strongest men are not those who sweat it out at work for long hours, but those who create their own set of values and judge their life by them.

Be honest at work

- Don't be afraid to tell your boss what you can and cannot do. If you think he or she is making unreasonable demands, say so. It's a sign of strength that your boss should respect.
- Saying you have a small problem early on can avoid a much big problem nearer a deadline.
- When you do have a large project to do, break it down into manageable chunks, and delegate work wherever possible.
- If you have subordinates, endeavour to motivate them. Encourage them to take part in unfamiliar tasks and to accept greater responsibility. Congratulate them on their successes.

Break time

Learn to appreciate the benefits of relaxation and leisure time. Try to take proper lunch breaks and get away from your desk as often as possible. If you spend your break only thinking about how to solve work-related problems, you're not getting the rest you need. Regular holidays are vital. Even if they're only for a few days, try to make the breaks completely restful. Resist calling the office unless it's absolutely necessary. Few of us are indispensable and holidays are for resting and recharging the batteries. A proper break will leave you fired up for when you return to work to face the next onslaught.

Learning to relax

Relax, don't do it – that is take on more work, get in an argument, or kick the cat. Knowing when and how to relax is the best antidote to stress. The cat will be happier, too.

Relaxation exercises

There are some simple tension-control exercises that can help you reduce the impact of stress:

- **Breathing deeply** Take a deep breath and exhale. Repeat this four or five times every two hours.
- **Meditate** If possible try to find a place to be alone during the day to collect your own thoughts. This could be on the stairs or even in a toilet cubicle.
- **Wait** If your morning drive to work leaves you stressed, spend a few minutes to compose yourself before getting out of the car.
- **Stretch** Move away from your desk to do a few simple stretches. And don't worry about what your colleagues think. Stretch arms, legs, and back, and roll your head. We store a lot of tension in our shoulders. Scrunch them up to your ears, keeping your head level, and release.

Laugh until you relax

- Laughter is the best medicine, which probably explains why comedians are the new pop stars. Joking aside, perhaps we can learn from the fact that children laugh 400 times a day on average, while adults only manage a derisory 15 laughs a day.
- When adults forgo play and focus exclusively on work, the resulting stress often leads to a variety of symptoms, including anxiety and muscular pain.
- When you laugh, chemicals are released into the brain called endorphins, which help to relax muscles and relieve pain.
- Of course, some situations you can't control. But try to use humour to defuse difficult situations and tense, uncomfortable atmospheres. After all, it's better to crack up laughing with others than to cry alone.

Top ten tips to help you relax

1. **Breathe deeply** Inhale through your nose, hold your breath for 10 seconds, then exhale. You should feel your stomach expand with each breath.

2. **Laugh** Make it a really big laugh; one of those ones that starts in your belly and surges through you almost out of control. Obviously, this can't be done to order. Go to a comedy night or watch a favourite TV comedy video. Failing that, laugh at a friend whose football team is mired in a relegation zone.

3. **Let go of negative thoughts** Try to banish work matters when you leave the office. If you really can't stop your brain churning through work problems, sit down and make a quick list of them to take to the office in the morning. Then stop worrying about them.

4. **Meditate or paint** Try to lose yourself in some form of spiritual activity on a regular basis. This will help to put your place in the universe in perspective.

5. **Relax all body parts** Relax each part of your body, starting with your feet. Do this by focusing all your thoughts on relaxing your toes. When your toes feel relaxed, shift your focus to your ankles, legs, and so forth up to your head.

6. **Stretch** Get up and stretch out to break physical tension. Stand up and leave your desk, and roll your head gently.

7. **Head rub** Place your fingers and thumbs on your scalp, apply as much pressure as is comfortable, and massage gently.

8. **Pick on a pillow** Pound a pillow to release tension, or scream into one to release pent-up pressure. It won't mind.

9. **Soak** Indulge yourself with a long soak in a warm bath.

10. **Enjoy** Find an activity that you like. It can be sedentary, such as writing or surfing the internet, or energetic, like cycling or running. Don't choose anything related to work.

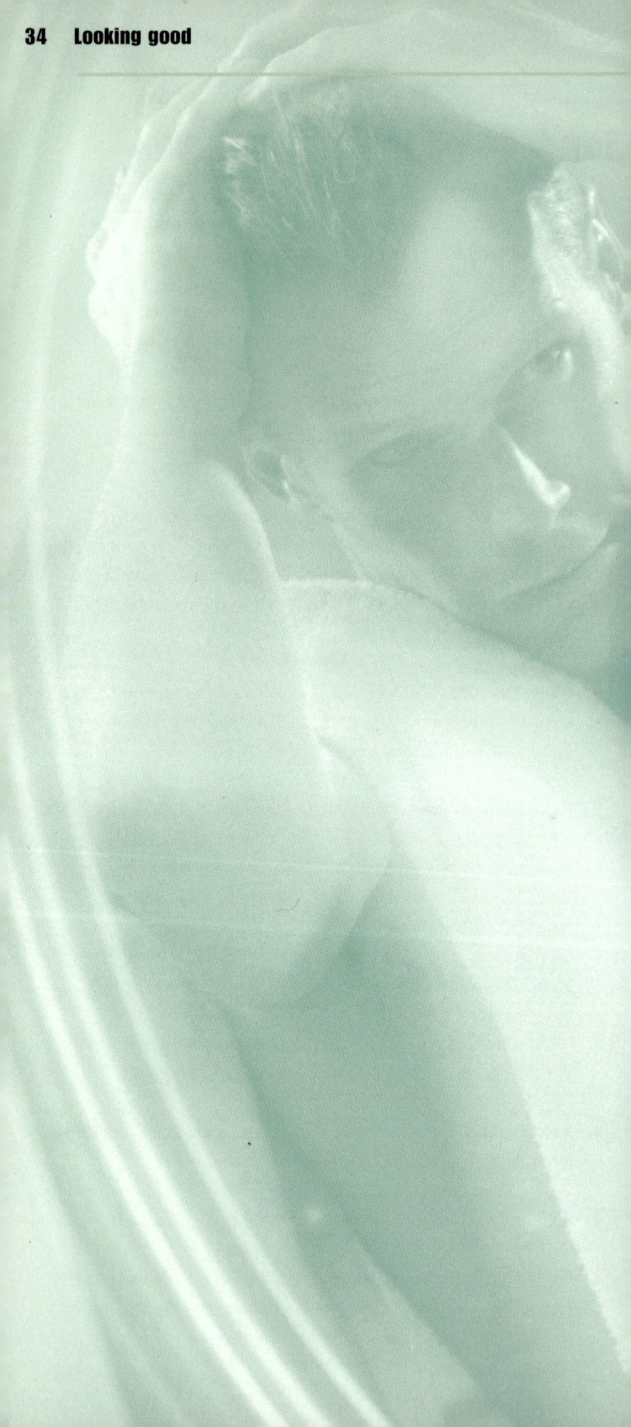

Looking good

Smooth and sexy skin
Healthy hair
Stylish hair
Dealing with hair loss
Hair elsewhere
Smelling fresh
Oral hygiene
Male nails

Smooth and sexy skin

If beauty is skin deep, why not look after your skin? It's waterproof, it renews itself, and it has erogenous zones. All it asks for is a little light maintenance.

Skin stats

- A square centimetre (⅙ square inch) of skin has about 600 sweat glands, 100 oil-secreting glands, 60 hairs, and countless nerve endings.
- The skin has three layers: from the top – the epidermis, which shows bruises; the dermis; and the subcutaneous layer.
- The top layer of skin sheds itself continually – an estimated 180kg (400lbs) of skin are shed over a lifetime.

Lotions and potions: are they just for girls?

Have you ever sneaked a dollop of moisturiser from your girlfriend's handbag? You're not alone. But nowadays you're just as likely to have your own. The cosmetics industry used to focus almost exclusively on women. But now many companies have seen a gap in the market and they've certainly plugged it. The array of products on the shelves today can be baffling, so here is a user's guide to what's on offer:

- **Soften up** Moisturisers can temporarily make skin look less dry and wrinkled because of the thin layer of oil that they leave on the skin. However, despite the claims, no products can reverse damaged skin or furrowed brows.
- **Soap and water** Washing your face with soap is fine for some men but if your skin is particularly dry, you might find soap leaves it feeling tight and flaky. Try using a facial wash instead, which replaces moisture rather than stripping it as soap does.
- **Unplug those pores** Exfoliating means using a facial scrub. Its grainy texture helps to get rid of dead skin, deeply ingrained dirt, and, most importantly, blackheads.

Ten top tips for great skin

1. **Shun the sun** The sun causes wrinkles. Wear a high-factor sun screen on all exposed skin and limit the amount of time that your skin is exposed – especially your face.

2. **Crow's feet** Got wrinkles around your eyes? This isn't about crows, but to do with sun and laughter. Creams containing alpha hydroxy acids (AHAs) may help fine lines, but expression lines are there to stay – and they add character.

3. **Feet first** Calluses and dead skin can build up on feet, especially if you play a lot of sport. Try a chiropody sponge or file to slough off dead skin.

4. **Less stress** Your skin will suffer if you are feeling stressed. Try to reduce stress levels with relaxation exercises.

5. **Health wealth** Don't smoke – it thins the skin and causes wrinkles. Drink alcohol in moderation. Eat plenty of fruit and vegetables, just like your mum told you. And drink at least six glasses of water a day.

6. **Clean up your act** Wash your face with soap or a facial wash. Use your hands because cloths and sponges may pull and rub your skin.

7. **Dry and flaky skin** Use a mild soap and apply moisturiser regularly. For mild eczema, use a product containing mainly water and glycerin.

8. **Oily problems** If your skin is on the oily side, avoid using fatted soaps or skin-softening emollients, which may give you whiteheads.

9. **Spot the difference** Acne affects 25 percent of men in their twenties and 10 percent in their thirties. Mild sufferers should use medicated hypoallergenic products. Consult a doctor if symptoms persist.

10. **Shelf life** Build up a store of moisturisers and lotions. Failing that, just rifle through your girlfriend's bathroom cabinet.

Know your skin

- All you need is a little understanding of what skin is to help keep it healthy. It consists of three layers. The thin, outer layer, the epidermis, is what you see. It's made up of dead cells that form a durable, waterproof surface. This is the layer that absorbs punishment from the sun, elements, and physical blows. It sheds itself constantly and is replaced by living cells below.
- The next layer, the dermis, is the thickest part of the skin. It contains a fibrous substance called collagen, which keeps the skin supple. It also contains hair roots (follicles), sweat and sebaceous glands, nerves, blood vessels, and fat.
- The smallest layer of skin is the subcutaneous fatty layer, below the dermis. Any product you apply to your skin, such as moisturiser, will do nothing to alter the chemistry of the living cells in the dermis, though it may temporarily plump up the outer layer of dead cells, making you look a little younger.

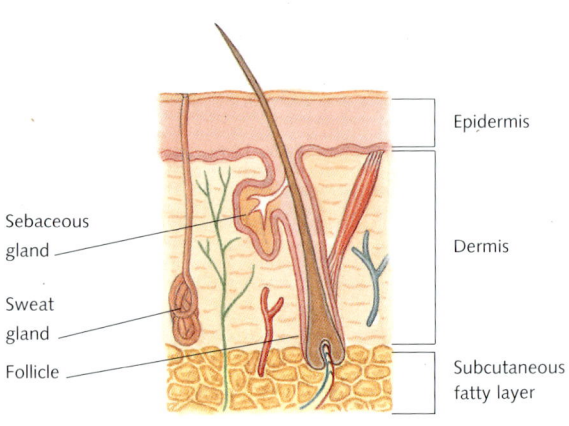

First aid for skin

Treat small cuts, scrapes, and minor burns with an over-the-counter antibacterial cream. Your chemist will advise you which one is best. For a mild case of sunburn, avoid spray-on products or creams. Instead, sit in a lukewarm bath and soak, then apply aftersun. Severe sunburn or any other kind of burn should be treated by a doctor.

Skin ailments

You might think your days of agonising over pimples would be a memory as distant as your first date. But oily skin can cause eruptions on a man's face well into his fifties. The major skin problems listed here should be diagnosed by your doctor:

- **Rosacea** This condition causes blood vessels to surface on the nose. Though no one knows why, this condition occurs more commonly in men. Rosacea is easily treated with topical creams and oral antibiotics.
- **Dermatitis** This is the generic name for skin inflammation. There are hundreds of such inflammations, including psoriasis and eczema. See a doctor if you have a recurring rash that doesn't respond to over-the-counter remedies.
- **Scars** Most cuts, especially small ones, heal without scarring. But larger wounds that aren't treated properly tend to leave scars. You can help to prevent scarring by never picking scabs. See your doctor if a wound is deep or jagged.

Adult acne

Remember when zits were the bane of your teenage life and stopped you chatting up the girl over the road or asking for a dance? Well for some men spots are an ongoing battle. About one in 100 men in their forties, for example, suffers outbreaks on the back, chest, and face. Whiteheads and other pimples may also continue to appear throughout life, depending on factors such as stress and oily skin. Acne appears when an oily gunk called sebum (secreted by sebaceous glands in the dermis) plugs up pores around hair follicles. Bacteria starts to grow and the pores become infected. There is no scientific support for the widely-held view that certain foods, such as chocolate, chips, and crisps, encourage acne. For severe causes of acne, you should consult your doctor. You may be prescribed antibiotics or a medication containing benzoyl peroxide, especially if you have oily skin. Always resist the temptation to squeeze pimples – you could make the infection worse and even cause scarring.

Healthy hair

Your hair is said to be the window to how healthy you are. Women say lank hair is a big turn-off. So brush up on the facts and banish those bad hair days.

General care

Whether you've got lots of hair or increasingly little, you can keep your tufts in good condition by:
- Getting a good cut every four to six weeks – this will keep the style in shape and stop the ends from drying out
- Washing and conditioning your hair regularly
- Using an appropriate styling product, such as a mousse or gel, to keep your hair looking good throughout the day

Stay in to wash your hair

Shampoo tips
You should shampoo frequently, unless your scalp is very dry. Regular washing will make your hair look fuller and will keep dandruff at bay. Use a mild shampoo – look for phrases such as "low pH" on the label. Harsher products will leave your hair dry and brittle.

When to condition
Even if you have very short hair you should use a conditioner once a week. This frequency is about right for men with fine or oily hair. But if you spend a lot of time in the sun or on the beach, you may need to use a deep conditioner every other day to combat dryness. How much you use and how often depends. If your hair seems too limp, use less, and if your hair seems too dry, use more.

Care with drying
Use the towel gently when drying your hair. Excessive tugging damages hair and can cause split ends.

Holding a style
Mousse is good for longer, wavy hair, while gels are better for shorter hair. But be aware that such products can build up in your hair, leaving it dull and limp. Use a clarifying shampoo once a week to strip away the build-up.

Hair care product guide

- Some dermatologists believe any shampoo will do, but many professional hair stylists disagree. They say that cheaper products are less effective and can leave your hair dry and duller in colour. If you have the cash, it's generally better to buy the more expensive hair care products that have gentler, less astringent contents.
- Try looking for products that contain only natural ingredients. Ask your barber or hairdresser for advice or visit a hair salon supply shop. Most manufacturers offer a range of products to suit all hair and scalp types, from dry to oily and fine to thick, and for those with dandruff or colour treatments.
- Shampoos are basically detergents for hair. A clarifying shampoo should be used occasionally to wash away any build-up of gel or mousse. Always use a mild shampoo with a low pH (acid-alkaline) balance.
- A conditioner makes brittle or dry hair soft. Fine hair needs a weekly conditioning, while coarse, dry hair needs more regular conditioning.
- Gels and mousses are used to give hard-to-manage hair style and body. Gel is heavier than mousse and better for shorter, fine hair. Avoid brands that contain alcohol as these can dry hair.

Hair and diet

- As with most aspects of the human body, a well-balanced and nutritious diet should be sufficient to keep your hair looking good.
- Protein plays a major role in the growth of hair and of nails. Proteins are essentially made up of amino-acids, which are instrumental in the building of new cells, including the cells that govern hair growth. Fish, seafood, poultry, and lean meat are all good sources of protein.
- Eating foods rich in vitamins and minerals will also encourage good hair growth.
- You should also be aware that some anti-malarial tablets, which have to be taken for prolonged periods before, during and after travelling, cause hair loss.

Stylish hair

Matching hair style to face shape

If you want more than just a haircut you should look beyond your usual barber and consider seeing a professional stylist. He or she will be able to create the right cut for you – one that matches your hair's texture, colour, and style with your facial structure. A good style should also be easy to care for. Here's a range of face shapes and styles that suit them:

Square
A good style to suit a square face is wide on top, flat at the sides, and perhaps keeps the hair slightly longer at the back.

Triangle
A triangular face is widest at the jaw and narrowest at the forehead. A good style for this shape is full at the top and narrower through the sides.

Heart
The cut should draw the eye away from the narrow chin, maybe through being left fuller in the back or with the addition of a fringe. Keep the parting off-centre.

Diamond
Go for a cut that's fuller in the back to offset the narrow chin. Part off-centre to disguise a narrow forehead.

Round
There are two contrasting styles to choose from if you have a round face: one is long yet narrow at the sides to add height; the other is cut close all over.

Oblong
Suitable hairstyles include a layered cut with full sides and a flat top.

Pear
For those with a pear-shaped face, your ideal hair cut should give fullness to the top and breadth to the forehead. A fringe can create the illusion of width.

Sharp rectangle
Try asymmetrical styles that widen the face. A fringe works well. Leave the sides full, with the back short.

Live and let dye

- An increasing number of men are now discreetly having their hair dyed using a process called weaving. The dye is woven through the hair to give the illusion of highlights so natural-looking that no one suspects dying.
- Alternatively, there are many do-it-yourself products available in the shops, but always follow the directions on the packet. Bleaching is the harshest of the hair-altering treatments as it sucks the colour out of the hair. Be aware that bleach is caustic and can damage skin, scalp, and eyes.

What about greying?

- There's little you can do to stop the onset of grey hair because melanin, the substance that gives hair its colour, diminishes with age. Your hair will naturally lose colour and turn whiter as you get older.
- Colouring your hair is the best disguise. You can try a do-it-yourself kit at home, but a professional stylist will probably do a better job and blend in the new colour more naturally.
- Other strategies are to boldly shave your head or, more simply, just to give in and keep your grey hair well groomed.

Top tips for choosing a stylist

- **Ask friends** Get friends whose hairstyles you like to recommend stylists.
- **Ask questions** Visit a likely barber shop or hair salon and find out how much experience they have.
- **Check responses** Go for a stylist who asks you about what you like and don't like and asks for suggestions. Does your stylist listen to you or does he or she seem to have a fixed idea about how it should be done?
- **Relax** Pick someone you feel relaxed with. A good stylist will make you enjoy your trip to the hairdresser's.
- **Stick with it** Once you've found a good stylist, stick with them – they can be rare. That way you'll build up a rapport, and you need never suffer the embarrassment of a bad hair cut again.

Dealing with hair loss

Hair today can soon become gone tomorrow. For many of us, hair loss is genetically inevitable. But there are ways to revitalise what you've got and make hair loss less apparent.

Folically challenged?

- Hair is formed from a protein called keratin and grows from follicles in the skin. The root (the only live part of the hair) grows and replaces dead hair with a new stand regularly.
- Men naturally lose 30–100 hairs a day through this natural process. Hair loss only becomes noticeable when you shed more than 200 hairs a day for several months.
- This can be triggered by a number of factors, including stress, illness, scalp infections, drugs or just natural, genetically pre-determined hair loss.

Male-pattern baldness

The biggest cause of hair loss is male-pattern baldness. This is genetically determined, so you can blame your father. Chemical receptors in the hair follicles convert testosterone (the male sex hormone) to dihydrotestosterone. This chemical causes the follicles to produce thin, downy hair that fails to cover the scalp.

What you can do

- If you find it impossible to grudgingly accept your personal "Millennium Dome", you have three choices: you can disguise it; you can have micrograft transplants; or you can use drugs.
- A little bit of good styling can do much to camouflage hair loss and this is definitely the cheapest option. Consider soft body waves and weaves as they add volume and texture to thinning hair by giving the appearance of more hair than there really is.
- Men with extensive loss might consider buying a custom-made hairpiece. Note the "custom-made". Unless you're a struggling comedian cheap, mass-produced wigs will only make people laugh.

Replacement treatments

- Hair replacement treatments have become increasingly popular as a way to permanently regrow hair. But be warned, regaining a realistic head of hair is expensive and there's little available in the UK that really works.
- Minoxidil, marketed as Regaine, is a drug that encourages regrowth in about one-third of men who try it. It seems to work best on men who are just starting to lose hair or those with fine hair, especially at the front. It's not intended for completely bald spots or for the "monk's circle".

If all else fails...

- The oral drug Propecia is freely-available in the US, but it's not licensed in the UK and must be obtained privately on a named-patient basis only, making it extremely expensive. In trials, however, it has been shown to stop hair loss and even stimulate regrowth. As with Minoxidil (see above) Propecia must be used permanently if it's to be effective.
- All balding men retain their remaining hair in a horseshoe pattern from the temples to the collar. If you're balding, resist the temptation to glue long, thin strands across your pate – you've never looked like Bobby Charlton on the football pitch and you don't want to look like him off it. Trying to cover your forehead up in this way only accentuates the bald parts and causes amusement at your expense.
- To make the most of what you've got left, keep your hair short. If you've got enough hair left, a soft body wave or a weave that adds colour will fill out your hair and add texture. A good stylist can also suggest suitable hair care products.
- The popular modern alternative is to shave off all your hair. If you do, you are no longer likely to be called Kojak but more likely to be regarded as trendy, hard, and sexy – consider Grant from Eastenders.
- A closely-shaved head might be the perfect option for you if you're reluctant to go completely bald.

Hair elsewhere

In a survey, nine out of ten men said they would prefer not having to shave their whiskers. Shaving's a bind. But a good shave can set you up with confidence for the day.

Shaving facts

- A wet shave undoubtedly gives the closest shave, but it's also more likely to lead to nicks, cuts, and skin irritation.
- Electric shavers are best for men with chronic ingrown hairs or any other skin malady, such as acne.
- Unlike a wet shave, an electric shave does not remove the top layer of skin. This reduces the likelihood of nicks but does not produce the smooth, fresh face feel of a wet shave.
- If you use an aftershave, choose one without alcohol to avoid stinging and dryness.
- Use a moisturiser or face-protecting cream especially produced for men to use after shaving to prevent your skin from drying out.

Electric or wet ?

WET
- A razor gives a much closer shave
- It takes longer but the benefits last longer
- Requires a good shaving gel or cream to soften the bristles
- Hard water does not lather as easily as soft
- It cannot be hurried
- Requires a very sharp blade
- The better razors can be quite expensive

ELECTRIC
- Electric shavers are more convenient and easier to use
- They work best on a clean, dry face
- They can be operated straight off the mains or charged up for portable use
- They don't require shaving cream or water
- They're less likely to cause nicks or ingrowing hairs

Top tips for the perfect shave

1. **Soften up** Ideally have a shower or bath before you shave to soften the hairs. Or you could try shaving in the bath!

2. **Warm water** Drench your face in warm, but not hot, water.

3. **Avoid soap** Use a shaving gel to apply a lather. Avoid using soap as this will dry your skin out over time.

4. **Take care** Hold your skin taut ahead of the razor and shave carefully in the direction of the whiskers' growth.

5. **Rinse and dry** Rinse your face with cold water, then apply a cold wet face cloth for about a minute. Dry your face and apply aftershave.

Avoid getting nicked

Nicks are unavoidable from time to time, especially when you're in a hurry. Who hasn't overslept and wielded the razor like a scythe? The problem is that the skin is covered in minute bumps and pimples. When the razor passes over them, it shaves off the tops, leaving you a bloody mess. Reduce your chances of getting nicks by lathering your face thoroughly, and remember to avoid shaving existing scabs and blemishes. A moisturising aftershave can also help your skin settle down.

Ingrown hairs

Curly-haired men suffer most from ingrown hairs. The hair starts to grow in a curled shape in the follicle and this makes it difficult to determine how to shave with the grain. When you shave, the skin can become inflamed and irritated, aggravating the ingrown hair and sometimes causing infection. If this causes severe pain, see a dermatologist.

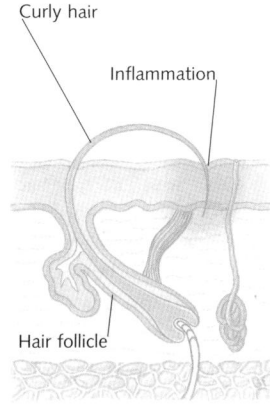

The ultimate beard

If you're growing a beard you should realise that certain types of beard suit certain face shapes. Below is an essential guide to which beards suit what shapes. But beards aren't for everyone. If you're still teased for having an angelic face, it's probably best to leave it on display. Men with fine hair and sporadically sprouting hair should also generally avoid beards.

Choosing a suitable style

A full beard and moustache look best on a narrow face, while a lean beard and moustache are most suitable on a round face. A beard that is unconnected to a moustache goes well with rounder faces, and round or square faces look good with a goatee and moustache. A standard beard and moustache look best on an oval face. Here are some beard variations to consider:

- **The beatnik** In fashion in the 1950s, the beatnik is similar to the goatee – a pointed tuft of hair on the end of the chin.
- **The Vandyke** Named after the 17th-century Flemish artist, the Vandyke is a longer, more pointed goatee than the Beatnik.
- **The Abraham Lincoln** This style has become less full and square than the more traditional beard worn by the American president.
- **The Elvis Presley** In his later Las Vegas years, Elvis wore mutton-chop sideburns trimmed at the jaw line, leaving his chin bare and giving the effect of a beard.
- **The ZZ Top** Long, flowing beards down to the waist are this group's trademark. Not recommended if you work with a lathe.
- **The Soul Patch** The actor Val Kilmer made the soul patch popular in his role as the frontiersman in the film Tombstone. He wore the patch – a small area of hair – on the chin just below the bottom lip.
- **The André Agassi** Popular among sportsmen and those in the entertainment industry, this full beard looks like stubble. It conveys a sense of casualness.

Beard maintenance

- A beard is like a vintage car – it can attract a lot of attention, but it requires a fair amount of maintenance.
- Most beards should be trimmed twice a week, preferably when the hair is dry. An electric beard trimmer does the best job. After the trim, you should tidy up the outlines of the beard. Using the length attachment, trim the edges of the beard from the bottom to the top.
- Beards should be washed, conditioned, and brushed daily. If your beard becomes cakey, wash it with a dandruff shampoo until it becomes soft again.
- To avoid infection, wash your beard accessories in shampoo periodically, and avoid borrowing or lending.

Nose and ear hair

Hair is prone to start sprouting out in new places from around age 40 – particularly in the ears and nose. Trim this tell-tale hair back with a pair of nail scissors, or ask a member of your family to buy you a special ear and nose trimmer for Christmas – they're bound to find it amusing. Nose and ear hair can also be removed permanently by electrolysis. This is a safe treatment that kills the hair follicles with jolts of electricity.

Beating body hair

A lot of men complain about excessive back and chest hair. There are a few options available to deal with it and here are some key factors to consider:

- Shaving body hair can cause ingrown hairs, stubbly, coarse regrowth of once-fine hairs, and five o'clock shadow.
- Depilatories are chemicals that dissolve fine hairs, but may leave behind coarse ones. They can burn if used incorrectly.
- Tweezing involves plucking hairs out individually.
- Waxing is like tweezing on a massive scale. A skin care specialist covers a small area in warm wax, allows it to harden and cool, then rips it off, tearing out unwanted hair with it.

Smelling fresh

No doubt you laughed at stink bombs in the playground. But what if it's now you who stinks in the office? You may be getting right up people's noses, so here are some facts to consider about personal hygiene.

What's that smell?

- Good smells are good but bad smells are awful. And the trouble is, body odour is so embarrassingly awful that it's the last thing people will tell you about.
- Secretions from your sweat glands are actually odourless. What makes them smell is the bacteria that multiply in the sweat. The strongest odour comes from the armpits and genitals where the apocrine glands (sweat glands in hairy parts of the body) secrete a milky fluid on which smelly bacteria thrive.

Aftershaves and colognes

The secret is to find a fragrance that suits your lifestyle and environment. Musk, for example, conveys sensual and sexy, which may not be appropriate for meeting the vicar. For the office, try something light, such as a citrus smell, and leave more sultry fragrances for the evenings. Other popular scent types include woody, spicy, and fruity fragrances. Try a few alternatives before buying one.

Sexual chemistry

Pheromones are natural chemical attractants used by many animals to meet and mate. In humans, too, there is evidence to suggest that pheromones play a part in sexual attraction. They are secreted under the armpits and in the genital area, and their impact may be diminished by daily washing. But remember, there's a thin line between smelling naturally sexy and naturally stinky.

Beating odours

- The best way to stay clean is to bath or shower daily. If you sweat a lot, shower more often.
- Daily bathing with a deodorant soap is usually sufficient, but avoid using this soap on your face as it can leave a residue and dry out your skin.
- Avoid scrubbing too hard as this can irritate the skin, and, in turn, encourage the growth of bacteria.
- If you're overweight, make sure you wash inside the folds of fat. Obesity can aggravate body odour.
- Watch out for spicy or fishy foods as they can attract the attention of bacteria on your skin.

Top tips for smelly feet

Your feet have more sweat glands than your armpits. The moisture they produce, combined with the dark warmth of your shoes, is a haven for millions of smelly bacteria.

1 **Kill the bacteria** If you've got a chronic foot odour problem, wash your feet every day with an antibacterial soap.

2 **Keep dry** Dry your feet thoroughly, especially between your toes, before putting on socks and shoes.

3 **Use preparations** Try foot powders, antiperspirants, and deodorants.

4 **Go natural** Wear natural fibre socks and get into the habit of using deodorant shoe inserts.

5 **Leather is best** Leather shoes allow your feet to breathe.

Masking odours

Antiperspirants work by reducing sweating by up to 40 percent. The active ingredients react with your sweat to form a gel that partially blocks sweat pores. Deodorants don't reduce sweating, but instead mask the odour with a mild perfume. They also contain chemicals that slow bacterial growth.

Oral hygiene

You can look clean, smart, and handsome, but if she keels over as soon as you open your mouth you haven't got a chance. What you need are some fresh air facts.

What causes bad breath?

- Bacteria on the tongue. About 90 percent of chronic bad breath is caused by a build-up of smelly bacteria at the back of the tongue where many people forget to brush.
- Gum disease. Diseases, such as gingivitis and periodontitis, can cause bad breath. The gums become red, soft, and swollen, and they often bleed. The problem can be caused by a large build-up of plaque and tartar at the gum line.
- Tooth decay. The decay is caused by plaque build-up.
- Food fragments. Pieces of food stuck between teeth cause plaque and tartar – ripe for attack by odour-producing bacteria.
- Plaque. This is a combination of food particles, bacteria, and saliva. In an unhealthy mouth, an overabundance of plaque decreases saliva, leaving you with a dry mouth and bad breath.
- Tartar. This is a hard substance that sticks between gums and teeth. It's what plaque turns into when you don't brush or floss adequately.
- Exhaled breath. The breath from your lungs may be scented by cigarette smoke or by a fishy, onion-rich, or garlicky meal.

Gum disease

Gum disease is chronic inflammation and infection of the gums caused by genetic predisposition and poor dental hygiene. About 70 percent of all adult tooth loss is caused by it. Early warning signs include: red, swollen, or tender gums; bleeding while brushing or flossing; gums that pull away from the teeth; and bad breath. There may be no discomfort or pain until the disease has spread so far that a tooth cannot be saved.

Top tips for fresher breath

1 Brush your teeth at least twice a day, preferably after every meal. Don't forget to floss.

2 Go for regular dental check-ups and visit a hygienist.

3 As an emergency measure, rinse your mouth with 225ml (8floz) of water mixed with half a teaspoon of salt.

4 A teaspoon of baking soda mixed with a glass of water makes a good home-made breath freshener.

5 Mouthwash, sugar-free mints, and breath fresheners only mask odour temporarily.

How to floss

Flossing is a vital part of dental hygiene as it removes plaque that a toothbrush can't reach. Dental tape is good if you have spaces between your teeth, waxed floss slides more easily, and spongy types are meant to fray less.

Wind half a length floss around one middle finger and the rest around the other. Move 3cm (1¼in) of floss gently between two teeth, then bend the floss around one tooth.

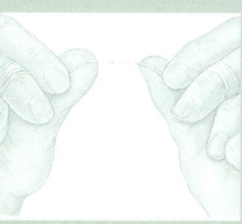

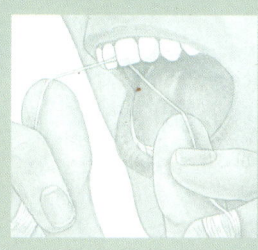

Slide the floss towards your gums and move the floss gently up and down. Remove the floss and unwind another piece from one of your fingers, then repeat the procedure with the next tooth.

Problem teeth

- The first rule of good dental health is to see a dentist at least once a year. Many men ignore their teeth until they have a serious problem, and by then it's too late. Dentists recommend having your teeth cleaned professionally at least twice a year.
- Plaque causes the two main problems – tooth decay and gum disease. If plaque is left it solidifies into tartar, which eventually penetrates the tooth's outer layer. If it reaches the inner layer, the pulp, you're looking at painful and expensive root-canal surgery. Stained teeth are a far less serious problem – ask your dentist about ways of whitening your teeth.

Know your teeth

- The external part of the tooth is divided into two parts, the crown and the root. The visible part of the tooth is covered with enamel. Beneath this is the dentine, which forms the largest part of the tooth. In the centre of the tooth is the pulp.
- Pulp contains nerves and blood vessels which enter the root of the tooth by the root canal. When an untreated cavity, fracture, or other injury exposes the pulp, bacteria will often seep in and cause an infection.

The best brushes

- Choose a toothbrush with a small head, about 2.5cm (1in) long, so that it's easy to move around.
- The bristles should be soft and nylon to avoid hurting your gums.
- Change your toothbrush every three to four months before the bristles become splayed. Old toothbrushes are ineffective and can harbour bacteria.
- Change your toothbrush after you've had an illness. The bacteria could be lurking in the brush.
- If you have manual dexterity problems, consider buying an electric toothbrush. There are plenty to choose from, and some models even have an alarm that lets you know when you've spent long enough on one part of your mouth. Ask your dentist for advice.

The best way to brush

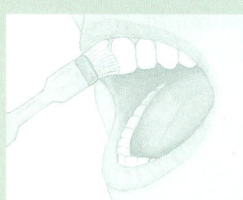
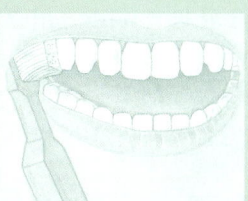

1. Place the brush head at a 45° angle against the gum line. Clean front teeth by moving the brush in small circles.

2. Brush the outer surface of upper and lower back teeth, keeping the brush at an angle against the gum line.

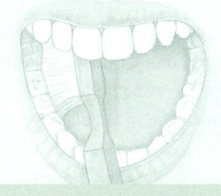
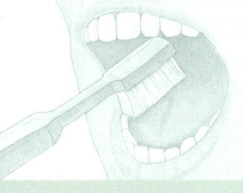

3. Clean the insides of the lower teeth, using small, circular movements and maintaining a 45° angle to the gum line.

4. Brush the biting surfaces of both the lower and upper teeth, using bold to-and-fro strokes.

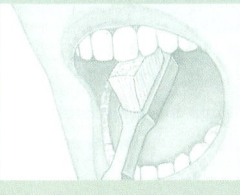

5. Use up-and-down strokes to clean the inner surfaces of the front teeth, tilting the brush vertically to make access easier.

Tooth-grinding

Some one in four people tooth-grind, which can lead to eroded teeth and jaw ache. Stress and tension are primary causes. Indications are: the tips of your teeth look flat; your jaw pops and clicks; and the enamel is worn. The best solution is to reduce your stress levels, or ask your dentist for a night guard.

Male nails

What is it with nails? Men hardly notice them, whereas women will be on cuticle alert as soon as they meet you. So keep them clean and get any problems nailed.

Nail grooming

- Nails are very easy to look after. The best thing is to keep them short by using nail scissors or clippers.
- Cut them in a curve, following the natural shape of your fingertips. Resist that curiously male tendency to use pen knives, paperclips and screwdrivers to do the job.
- Use a moisturiser to keep your nails and hands well tended. If your cuticles are white and cracking, use a heavy moisturiser until they soften up, otherwise a lighter moisturiser should do.
- If your nails are stained, put a few drops of regular laundry bleach in a bowl of water and washing-up liquid and scrub with a brush. Then apply moisturiser to avoid brittleness and cracking.

How to trim your nails

- The easiest time to cut your nails is after a bath or shower when they are at their softest.
- A well-trimmed fingernail has a small edge of white protruding over a rosy nail bed.
- Cut the nails straight across if your fingertips are squarish, or with a slight curve if they're curved, and only ever use nail clippers or scissors.
- If you end up with some sharp edges, use a nail file to smooth them off. File the nails from the corners to the centre. Filing from the centre to the corners can cause nails to flake and become brittle.
- Deal with nail splits quickly to prevent further damage.
- Keep a nail file at work and at home to smooth nicks and tears.
- Never cut cuticles or push them back too hard.

Problem nails

- **Hangnails** They're those slithers of dry skin that split from the cuticle of skin surrounding the nail and get snagged on your clothes. Trim them with nail scissors or clippers. Do not bite them, pull them, or tear at them. And avoid ripping out live skin as it can bleed or become infected.
- **Biting** If you bite your nails it's probably because you're stressed. The best solution is to buy chewing gum to bite on. Another option is to coat your nails in Stop 'n' Grow, a varnish that contains two very bitter chemicals.
- **Fungal problems** If your fingernails turn fungal, use an antibacterial soap to prevent infection. Over-the-counter antifungal creams can also be used if your nails turn green, or if a yellow or white spot grows larger over time. The worst fungal problems are usually in the toenails. Try drying your feet with a hairdryer and dusting your toes with antifungal powder. Wear shoes that allow your feet to breathe and do whatever you can to keep your feet clean and dry.
- **Blackened nails** Knocks and bruises cause nails to blacken when blood vessels under the nail plate break. Leave the nail alone and it will fall off of its own accord.

Top tips for neat nails

1. **Don't bite** Leave your teeth out of nail maintenance.

2. **Use the right kit** Only use nail scissors or clippers.

3. **Short is best** Unless you play guitar, keep your nails short.

4. **Prevent dryness** Apply hand lotion to dry or cracking cuticles. Dehydration can cause nails to chip or crack – apply petroleum jelly to the nails before going to bed.

5. **Stop smoking** Nicotine nails are a major turn-off.

6. **Remove stains** Yellow, stained nails can be cleaned. Soak them for 10 minutes in a solution of equal parts warm water and hydrogen peroxide. Then scrub gently with a nail brush.

7. **Eat a balanced diet** Protein is particularly important for nails.

The right diet

The right diet

Eating for life
Major food groups
Vital vitamins
Must-have minerals
The food pyramid
Planning what you eat
Weighty matters
Shedding the flab
Drinking to your health
Organic eating
Food supplements

Eating for life

Busy lives often mean that men leave their diets to chance. By learning the basics of good nutrition you should be able to enjoy good health – whether you're working late at the office or training for a marathon.

The right food

- Food provides the nutrients your body needs for survival and good health. There are six main nutrient groups – proteins, carbohydrates, fats, vitamins, minerals, and water. Fibre isn't a nutrient, but it is a very important part of a healthy diet.

- Each man's dietary requirements are unique and factors, such as lifestyle, body type, and genes, all determine nutritional needs. However, there are broad rules that should form the basis of all diets: eat plenty of fruit, vegetables, and grains; drink lots of water; and minimise your fat intake.

- The food pyramid (see p.68) tells you what foods to place at the heart of your diet, what to eat in moderation, and what to leave on the supermarket shelf. This is the starting point if you're going to take control of your eating habits.

- If you follow the food pyramid logic, chances are you'll have to part company with some old friends. Fatty and sugary foods will increase both your girth and your chances of getting heart disease, so prepare to ditch some of the following: meat, especially beef and pork products, dairy products, mayonnaise, biscuits, cakes, and doughnuts. If you have high cholesterol levels, it's particularly important to avoid too much saturated fat – found in animal products, including meat and eggs.

- Once you understand your nutritional requirements, you need to devise a game plan. Start by writing down the changes you want to make ("I want to eat less sugar and more complex carbohydrates"). Say why you want to make these changes ("Cut the risk of heart disease"), and write down achievable goals ("Eat fish instead of steak twice a week").

Nourishing facts

- Proteins help in the body's growth and repair of cells, muscles, and skin.
- Carbohydrates are burned for energy and keep skin, bones, and nails healthy.
- Fats are burned and also stored for future energy needs. They also insulate against heat loss.
- Vitamins regulate metabolism and are vital for growth, digestion, and reproduction.
- Minerals are inorganic substances that are involved in countless chemical processes.
- Water cools and lubricates the body and transports nutrients through the circulatory system. It flushes out waste and toxins.
- Fibre keeps the digestive tract clean and functioning well.

Common eating mistakes

- **Skipping breakfast** Start the day with a decent-sized breakfast consisting of cereal, skimmed milk, and fruit juice rather than artery-clogging bacon, egg, and sausages.
- **Eating too much fat** Saturated fat converts into cholesterol, which puts extra pressure on the heart.
- **Crash dieting** Quick-fix diets don't work in the long term.
- **Eating irregularly** Fasting for four to six hours or more lowers your blood sugar levels, leading to irritability and fatigue.
- **Drinking too much alcohol** Limit your consumption. More than three units a day can lead to addiction, illness, or accidents.

Instant ways to eat well

- **Take more fibre** It reduces cholesterol, protects you from colon cancer, and helps prevent irregular bowel function.
- **Snack away** Healthy snacking can help boost energy levels, but steer clear of chocolates and sweets. Instead go for fruit, wholemeal bread, and vegetable sticks.
- **Sleep empty** Don't eat just before bedtime as it's likely to cause insomnia, indigestion, or heartburn. Have only a light meal for supper and eat the day's main meal at lunchtime.
- **Go low-fat** Look for low-fat alternatives of your fatty favourites. If you eat beef or pork, for example, go for the leanest cuts available.

Major food groups

1. **Proteins** These complex molecules make up 15–20 percent of your body weight and provide the body's main building materials. When you digest food, your body turns the large protein molecules (from poultry, fish, and eggs, for example) into amino acids. These smaller molecules are then put back together again to form the main ingredients for the growth and repair of skin, bones, muscles, hair, teeth, and all other types of body tissue. Note that a high protein intake, perhaps including supplements, doesn't necessarily turn you into a muscleman. It does, however, provide the raw material if you are exercising at sufficiently high levels to build up muscle.

2. **Carbohydrates** These are found in sugars (refined sugar, honey, and treacle) and starches (vegetables, fruit, pulses, and whole grains). They are burned by the body at varying speeds to generate the energy needed for us to grow, repair ourselves, move around, and keep warm. Sugars are known as simple carbohydrates, because they are quickly digested into glucose (blood sugar), which is metabolised into energy by our muscles and organs. Starches are complex carbohydrates and are broken down into glucose and absorbed into our bloodstreams in a slower and more controlled manner. As well as providing energy, carbohydrates have other vital roles. They help to break up the fat that can lead to obesity and heart disease, and they contribute to the appearance and health of your skin, bones, and nails.

3. **Fats** Yes, as we all should know by now, too much fat-laden food can lead to increased waistlines and clogged arteries, but fat is still a vital component of your diet. It's burned as energy and stored for future use in case other energy sources run low. Fat teams up with proteins to form membranes (semi-permeable skins) around every cell. Fat also insulates the body from heat loss as it is laid down in layers beneath the skin. It cushions vital organs, such as the kidneys and liver, by growing in "pads" around them.

Where to find them

1 **Proteins** Fish, seafood, poultry, lean meat, and offal are all rich sources of proteins, since they are made from animal cells. Eggs and dairy products also contain proteins because in nature they are the natural products providing nourishment for the growth of animals. Beans, whole grains, maize, and nuts are also all rich in proteins, in addition to containing large amounts of complex carbohydrates. These foodstuffs are particularly important to vegetarians and vegans, as they will form their only source of protein. Between 50–110g (2–6oz) of protein foods should be consumed daily.

2 **Complex carbohydrates** These are generally found in the fleshy parts of vegetables, fruits, pulses, and grains. Foods, such as bread, pasta, rice, kidney beans, and avocados, all contain high levels of complex carbohydrates. They tend to be heavy and filling foods, and should make up to two-thirds of your daily food intake.
Simple carbohydrates These are characterised by their sweetness. Treacle, syrup, honey, and confectionery are all high in simple carbohydrates, and refined sugar is a pure source. They are good for instant energy, but should make up only a small fraction of your daily intake. They contain little nutritional value and also contribute to tooth decay.

3 **Fats** All fats derived from animal sources are saturated. Although the body will readily digest them, their intake should be kept to a minimum, because of the detrimental effects they can have if they start building up in the body. Palm and coconut oils are saturated, too.
Unsaturated oils are far more beneficial in the diet. Vegetable oils are polyunsaturated (partly saturated), while olive oil is monounsaturated. Olive oil is the most beneficial to the body. Because of the high levels of carbohydrates needed in your diet, fats and oils should only represent some 5 percent of your daily intake. Many men consume far in excess of this percentage.

Vital vitamins

Vitamins are only needed in relatively small quantities, but without them we begin to malfunction. Most vitamins cannot be produced by our bodies, so it's crucial that we include them in a healthy diet that features a wide variety of different foods.

Vitamin check list

WATER-SOLUBLE VITAMINS

- **Vitamin C** is an antioxidant necessary for building bones, forming neurotransmitters, which transmit electrical signals, and detoxifying the liver. It boosts immunity and helps prevent colds. **Good sources:** Oranges, grapefruit, red peppers, raw spinach, potatoes, broccoli, Brussels sprouts. **Daily requirement:** 60mg

- **Thiamin (Vitamin B_1)** helps convert carbohydrates to energy. Deficiency may cause fatigue and appetite loss. **Good sources:** Peas, beans, whole grains, pork. **Daily requirement**: 1.4mg

- **Riboflavin (Vitamin B_2)** helps create energy from food. Vital in the formation of red blood cells and hormones. Helps maintain tissues. **Good sources:** Milk products, whole grains, broccoli, asparagus, potatoes, oranges, eggs, liver. **Daily requirement:** 1.6mg

- **Niacin (Vitamin B_3)** helps create energy from food. **Good sources:** Grains, cereals, baked foods, meat, poultry, fish, peanuts, beer. **Daily requirement:** 18mg

- **Pantothenic acid (Vitamin B_5)** helps metabolise food and helps produce key hormones and neurotransmitters. **Good sources:** All animal and vegetable tissue. **Daily requirement:** 6mg

- **Vitamin B_6** helps regulate the nervous system. Important in breaking down protein and amino acids and converting them into energy. Also helps in the metabolism of glucose and fatty acids, and in the production of red blood cells. **Good sources:** Whole grains, potatoes, chicken, fish, egg yolks, bananas, avocados. **Daily requirement:** 2mg

- **Vitamin B_{12}** is essential for DNA synthesis, and cell production and division. **Good sources:** Liver, oysters, beef, pork, whole-milk dairy products, eggs. **Daily requirement:** 1mcg (microgram)

- **Folic acid** is required for the growth and division of cells and the formation of haemoglobin. **Good sources:** Beans, cereals, spinach, asparagus, broccoli, okra, various seeds, liver. **Daily requirement:** 200mcg

- **Biotin** helps immune system function. Vital in food metabolism and the formation of proteins, hormones, and neurotransmitters. **Good sources:** Peanut butter, pulses, nuts, grains, egg yolks, offal, yeast, cauliflower. **Daily requirement:** 0.15mcg

FAT-SOLUBLE VITAMINS

- **Vitamin A** is required for normal vision, reproduction, cell development, growth, and immunity. It maintains the health of the skin and membranes. Beta-carotene, which converts to vitamin A in the body, is an antioxidant. **Good sources:** Peaches, carrots, spinach, broccoli, tomatoes, lettuce, green beans, fish, liver, egg yolks, whole milk. **Daily requirement:** 800mcg

- **Vitamin D** is key to bone building, healthy teeth, and nerve-muscle interaction. **Good sources:** Sunshine, canned sardines, salmon, fortified dairy products. **Daily requirement:** 5mcg

- **Vitamin E** is an antioxidant. It lowers cholesterol and helps prevent a build-up of plaque in arteries. It boosts immunity, helps prevent cataracts, and may help prevent heart disease. **Good sources:** Nuts, sunflower seeds, green leafy vegetables, wheat germ, whole grains. **Daily requirement:** 100mg

- **Vitamin K** helps regulate blood clotting. **Good sources:** Green, leafy vegetables, fruit, seeds, eggs, dairy products, meat. **Daily requirement:** 60–80mcg

Must-have minerals

Minerals are not as specifically linked to particular foods as vitamins, so a less varied diet will usually provide them. You must aim for maximum variety, however, for the sake of your vitamin needs. The minerals listed below are the ones you need the most of.

Mineral check list

1. **Calcium** is key to building bones and teeth among other important roles. It may protect against high blood pressure and colon cancer. Good sources: Dairy products, sardines, broccoli, leafy vegetables. Daily requirement: 800mg

2. **Chloride** is another essential mineral, primarily for the nervous system and for maintaining fluid balance. Good sources: Table salt. Daily requirement: 300–400mg

3. **Magnesium** is a bone-builder that helps regulate the heart and protects against heart disease. Important in enzyme activity, and in metabolism. Good sources: Green leafy vegetables, pulses, seafood, nuts, soya beans, eggs, whole grains, dairy products. Daily requirement: 300mg

4. **Phosphorus** is vital for bone building, it helps maintain the body's fluid balance, and is important in metabolism. Good sources: Dairy products, meat, fish, grains, nuts, beans. Daily requirement: 800mg

5. **Potassium** regulates blood pressure and heart function. It's vital for muscle contraction and transmission of nerve impulses. Good sources: Citrus fruits, bananas, most other fruits and vegetables, seafood. Daily requirement: 3500mg

6. **Sodium** is also important in the transmission of nerve impulses, regulating blood pressure, and in metabolism. Good sources: Natural foods; added to many canned and frozen foods, cereals, and crisps. Daily requirement: 2400mg

Other diet essentials

Water – why we need it

• Water really is the elixir of life, for without it nothing could live. It serves many purposes in your body: it's a medium for carrying substances around the body; it provides the lubrication for your movements; and it holds your cells rigid.

• Good old H_2O absorbs the goodness from your digested food and carries waste away in your urine. It enables some men to shed tears and allows you to sweat. Water accounts for around 80 percent of your body mass, and you will die if you allow yourself to dehydrate by only a few percent.

• Water is obtained from drinks and food. It may seem unnecessary to remind someone to consume enough water, but some people do not register a thirst when they are dehydrating. It's also worth remembering that extreme perspiration, crying, and a runny nose can all lead to both dehydration and extreme cramps from the loss of salt in sweat, tears, and mucus. Heavy consumption of alcohol has a similar effect.

Fibre facts

• Fibre is not absorbed into the body at all. Nevertheless, it's vital for good health – helping you digest and preventing constipation.
• It's the material in plant food (vegetables, fruit, grains) that your body can't digest.
• Fibre gives a full feeling without the extra calories.
• It cleans the digestive tract as it passes along it.
• The recommended daily intake is 20–30g (³⁄₄ –1oz).

Sources of fibre

All-bran cereal (85g [3oz])	8.6g
Apple (with skin)	2.8g
Brussels sprouts (180g [6oz])	5.0g
Bread slice (wholemeal)	2.4g
Green peas (90g [3½oz])	5.4g
Kidney beans (85g [3oz])	6.9g
Lentils (85g [3oz])	5.2g
Orange (small)	2.9g
Potato (medium, baked)	5.0g
Spaghetti (140g [5oz], wholemeal)	5.4g

The food pyramid

Use the pyramid to check if you're consuming a variety of foods in the right proportions. Eat plenty of foods from the lower two tiers, but consume those near the top sparingly.

Level 1
Fats, oils, sugars

Level 2
Dairy products, animal and plant proteins

Level 3
Fruits, vegetables

Level 4
Grains, bread, cereal, pasta, rice, potatoes

Level 1
Fats, oils, sugars, sweets, and confectionery: ½–1½ daily servings. One serving = four teaspoons of sugar or oil, or two chocolate bars

Level 2
Dairy products and proteins: 4–6 daily servings. Serving = a mug of milk, 25g (1oz) hard cheese, 90g (3½oz) lean meat

Level 3
Fruits: 2–4 servings. One serving = a piece of fruit, or half a mug of fruit juice. Vegetables: 3–5 servings. Serving = a handful of raw vegetables, or half a mug of juice

Level 4
Grains, bread, cereal, pasta, rice, potatoes: 6–11 servings. Serving = medium bread slice, or half a bowl of cereal

Your own food processor

What happens to food after you eat? Before your body can use the food, it must be broken down and converted into substances in the digestive tract that your body can use.

STAGE 1 THE MOUTH
The thought of food will already have triggered the release of saliva and mucus in your mouth. Your teeth and tongue cut, mash, and mix the food, while chemicals in saliva help break it down before it's swallowed in small amounts.

STAGE 2 THE STOMACH
Hydrochloric acid and other gastric juices attack the food, and powerful muscle contractions churn it until it becomes a soupy liquid called chyme.

STAGE 3 THE SMALL INTESTINE
The liquid drains into the small intestine where it's met by enzymes secreted by the liver, pancreas, and gallbladder that finish digestion. This long intestine is coated with millions of hair-like structures called villi through which the food (now refined chemicals) is absorbed. These chemicals will travel to every cell in the body via the bloodstream and the highways of the lymph system.

STAGE 4 THE LARGE INTESTINE
Excess water and remaining useful minerals are absorbed back into the body through the large intestinal (or colon) wall. What is left passes into the rectum as faeces and leaves the body through the anus after several hours.

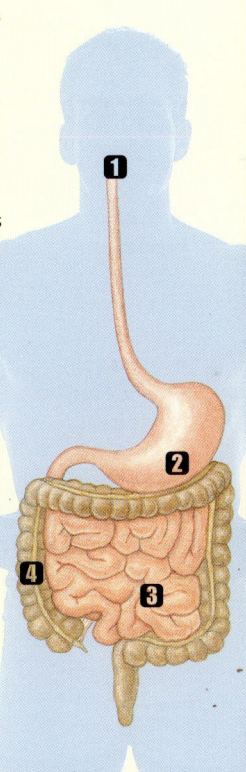

Planning what you eat

This chart lists examples from the four food groups in the food pyramid (p.68) in more detail so you plan the healthiest possible daily meals.

Menu planning guide

Food group	One serving	Serving tips
Grains, bread, cereals, pasta, rice, potatoes *(level 4)*	115g (4oz) potatoes, 90g (3½oz) pasta, rice etc., 25g (1oz) cereal	Use wholegrain bread and cereals when you can
Fruit and vegetables *(level 3)*	Large salad, 90g (3½oz) cooked vegetables	Include at least one citrus fruit or some berries
Lean cooked meat, fish or poultry, eggs, pulses (peas, beans, lentils), cheese with varying levels of fat content *(level 2)*	2 eggs, 150g (5oz) yogurt, 90g (3½oz) lean meat, fish, or poultry, 175g (6oz) pulses, 25g (1oz) hard cheese, 40g (1½oz) medium-fat cheese (Brie, Edam, ricotta), 115g (4oz) low-fat cheese	Combine pulses with cereals for a balanced intake of protein if you are vegetarian or vegan. Calcium-enriched soya milk is a highly nutritious alternative for people allergic to dairy produce
Fat and oils *(level 1)*	15–25g (½–1oz) butter, margarine, or refined oils	Use fats and oils sparingly for cooking and dressings

Top tips for balanced eating

1. Variety is best The best dietary advice is to eat as wide a variety of food as possible. This will enable you to consume the recommended daily allowances (RDAs) of all essential vitamins and minerals as well as the right amounts of proteins, carbohydrates, and fats.

The simplest way to do this is to eat foods from each of the four main food groups every day (see the food pyramid p.68). The group from which you should eat the most includes breads, cereals, grains, and rice; the second, fruits and vegetables; the third, dairy produce, animal proteins (such as fish, meat, poultry) and plant proteins (such as dried beans, peas, nuts, and seeds) and the group you should eat the least of includes fats, oils, and sugars.

Avoid eating too much of any one kind of food, as it can lead to weight gain. And don't become a complete slave to your diet. Food is one of life's social pleasures, so enjoy it.

2. Diet plus exercise Health is something many of us take for granted until we lose it. But maintaining a healthy diet and exercising regularly is a winning lifestyle formula. By being aware of specific risks to your health and alert to early symptoms of illness, you can hope not only to live longer but also to enjoy a better quality of life. This is not so difficult to achieve.

Some health factors, such as your genes, are cast in stone, but how much you smoke and drink, what you eat, and how often you exercise are things you can control. Many men consume too much fat, too many sugary foods, and too much beer. Cut down on them – they're a major source of weight gain. Instead, eat more fibre and drink plenty of water. Your body will thank you for it.

3. Food and fitness If you're overweight, regular physical activity will boost your metabolic rate so that you burn up more calories even at rest. It's true that the more active you are, the more calories you need, but you should obtain them readily from a balanced diet. The best types of food to eat before exercise are starchy carbohydrates, such as pasta and potatoes. Try to eat three hours or more before you work out, and drink lots of water to compensate for lost fluids.

Weighty matters

Not only is obesity a turn-off, it also has serious consequences for your health. Many of us are overweight today due to sedentary lifestyles and high-fat diets, but attaining a healthy weight is the greatest asset to health.

Are you overweight?

If you are more than 20 percent above your optimal body weight or wearing 25 percent body fat, you're at risk. Check how much you should weigh using the chart opposite.

Why does it matter?

If you fall within the danger zones it means you're more susceptible to high blood pressure, clogged arteries, strokes, heart attacks, and colon and prostate cancer.

Putting weight on

After age 30, a man's metabolic rate starts to slow down, which often leads to an average weight gain of 500–700g (18–25oz) a year.

What is cholesterol?

Cholesterol is a soft, fat-like substance, which the liver uses to help form cell membranes (semi-permeable skins) and hormones (chemical messengers). Cholesterol is produced by the liver and much of it comes from our food. If you consume too many foods rich in saturated fats you'll have more cholesterol than your body needs. Excess cholesterol clings to artery walls as fatty deposits, which can eventually cause blockages. Such obstructions can, in turn, lead to heart attacks and strokes. If you have a history of heart disease or high cholesterol in your family, get a cholesterol check at your doctor's surgery.

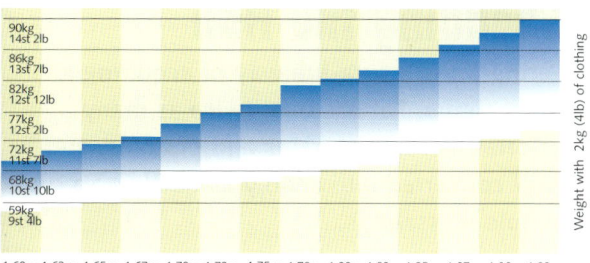

Top three causes of weight gain

1. **Eating too much** Most of us eat more food than our bodies actually need. If you eat more calories than you burn, the excess gets converted into fat, which is stored in fat cells.

2. **Lack of exercise** If you want to burn off excess calories and avoid getting fat, you need to exercise. Get off your butt if you want to lengthen your lifespan.

3. **Fat genes** It's not entirely your parents' fault, but you are genetically programmed to carry a certain amount of fat. It's no excuse for lack of exercise though.

Draw a line from your weight on the left to your waist size on the right. The point where the line intersects the central scale will give you an estimate of your body fat percentage.

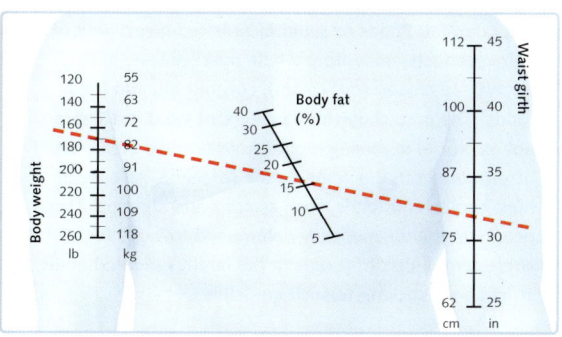

Shedding the flab

Eating fat is a sure-fire way of acquiring a fuller figure. Fat has over twice as many calories as carbohydrates and proteins, and it isn't converted into energy as quickly. So the simple message is...

Eat less fat

Cutting fat from your diet is the key to weight loss. Experts say that you should get only 5 percent of calories from fat, and if you want to lose weight you should be aiming for even less than this. Eat more complex carbohydrates, such as vegetables, fruit, wholemeal bread, and pulses. Not only do they provide lots of minerals and vitamins, but they are also fat burners as your body has to work harder to digest them.

Do more exercise

Just cutting back on fat will not make you lose weight. Exercise is missing from the equation. Aerobic exercise (sustained, rhythmic exercise using large body muscles) steps up the rate at which your body burns fuel. Try 30 minutes of jogging, cycling, swimming, football, or tennis three times a week.

Cutting cholesterol

To lower your cholesterol levels limit your intake of saturated fat. Foods to avoid include red meat, pork, dairy products made from whole milk (cheese, butter, yogurt, ice cream, sour cream), coconut oil, and fried foods. The pure cholesterol content of what you eat is not as crucial in raising blood cholesterol as the levels of saturated fat. But to be on the safe side, go easy on high-cholesterol foods, such as eggs and shrimps. Those people that are genetically determined towards high cholesterol levels (if it runs in the family) should be very strict about sticking to such guidelines.

Top ten tips for fat fighting

1. **Slash and burn** The only way to melt excess blubber in the long term is to burn more calories than you consume. That's why you need long-term strategies, such as cycling instead of driving to work, and switching to low-fat milk.

2. **Crash diets** Crash diets don't work even if you can bear the regimes. Your metabolism slows down when you stop eating and takes a while to return to normal when you start again.

3. **Fat substitutes** Learn to live without high-fat favourites by substituting them with tasty alternatives. Sorbet instead of ice cream, for instance, or dried apricots instead of peanuts.

4. **Don't torture yourself** If you push too hard to curtail fat, you'll just get frustrated and switch back. It's still OK to eat ice cream – just not every day.

5. **Packed lunches** If the canteen's lunchtime special is stodge and chips, why not take in your own low-fat lunch? Maybe pack a lean chicken sandwich and always include fruit.

6. **Night pickings** Your digestive capacity drops by 20–40 percent at night, and when you go to bed you're not exercising to burn it off (well not all night).

7. **Savour the flavour** It takes about 20 minutes for your body's feedback system to realise you've had enough food. If you eat too quickly you'll unwittingly eat more than you need.

8. **Read the labels** The nutritional information panels on food packets give details about fat and calorie contents. Use them to make informed choices about what you eat.

9. **Cut back on booze** If you're trying to lose weight, cut out booze. Alcoholic drinks contain calories with little nutritional value but plenty of potential to expand your waistline.

10. **Lighten the dessert** When you're craving something sweet after your main course go for something light and non-fatty, like a nice, crunchy apple which has no fat and few calories.

Drinking to your health

All hail to the ale and a cheer for the beer! Yes, alcohol is great, but only if you drink a sensible amount. Science tells us that moderate drinkers have healthier hearts and live longer than heavy drinkers and teetotallers.

Booze benefits

Not only does moderate drinking help you relax and give you a mild sense of euphoria, it can also help to prevent heart attacks and strokes. Alcohol increases your levels of HDL cholesterol, which helps carry away the artery-clogging LDL cholesterol. It also decreases the blood's ability to form clots.

And the bad news...

Medical research has shown that if you cross the line from moderate drinking all the positive effects go down the tube. Instead of preventing heart disease, drinking can actually cause it by raising the risk of heart attacks and strokes by damaging heart muscles and raising blood pressure.

Heavy drinking problems

- Drinking too much alcohol has implications for every organ in your body. Brain cells are destroyed, nerve damage can lead to impotence, and toxins damage sperm. Liver cancer or cirrhosis may develop, and digestion is impaired. Alcohol abuse also gives rise to a range of social problems. Half of all traffic deaths, for example, and at least a quarter of murders and suicides are alcohol related.
- The effects of drinking differ widely between individuals, but at some point the ill effects of too much drink will concern everybody. While moderate drinkers experience feelings of relaxation, exhilaration, and increased sexual desire, heavier drinkers may experience hangovers, disrupted sleep, slurred speech, memory lapses, impaired judgement, and depression – as well as the health problems listed above.

Top five hangover cures

While we may not realise the long-term damage drinking too much alcohol does to our bodies, we all know what the short-term consequence is – the dreaded hangover. You might not be able to eliminate nausea, dizziness, and a pounding headache, but you'll be able to make the morning after more bearable if you follow these tips:

1. **Fruit juice** A glass of orange juice will help speed the removal of any remaining alcohol in your bloodstream.

2. **Pain relief** To alleviate headaches take a mild pain reliever, such as paracetamol or aspirin.

3. **Drink water** Two or three glasses of plain water will hinder dehydration – one of the causes of a hangover. Try to drink two to three glasses before you go to bed.

4. **Vitamin C** Take a supplement, or eat fruit that's rich in vitamin C, such as oranges, grapefruit, and strawberries.

5. **Be patient** The only thing that really heals a hangover is time. In about 24 hours you'll feel a lot better.

Safe limits

The benefits of alcohol depend on moderation. For most men that means no more than three units of alcohol a day. (A unit is defined as a half pint of beer or one glass of wine.) The limit for men endorsed by the British Medical Association is 21 units a week, but many men drink more than this. There are other ways you can make drinking safer as well as unit watching. Eat something first as food in the stomach slows absorption and reduces the severity of hangovers. Drink more slowly – try and make one drink last an hour. Don't drink every day otherwise you'll build up a tolerance and drink more. Alternate alcoholic with non-alcoholic drinks and leave the bubbly for special occasions because fizzy drinks are absorbed faster into the bloodstream.

Organic eating

With growing evidence that farming pesticides can cause cancer and other health problems, many people want a choice in what they eat. Organic foods still cost a bit more, but they're safer and tastier.

What's the difference?

- The 20th century saw the agrochemical industry expand to such an extent that artificial plant food yields – in the West at least – made food shortages a thing of the past. But the use of chemicals to achieve this has prompted growing disquiet.
- Critics point to the spraying of more than 200 chemicals on our food crops as a cause of cancer, allergies, birth defects, and other health problems. A recent survey found pesticide residues in almost all types of food and even in mothers' milk.
- Organic farming means more than just farming without chemicals. It has the broader aim of developing techniques for fostering healthy, fertile soil through the sensitive management of crops. Organic food is free from genetically modified products, agrochemical residues, and artificial preservatives.

Genetically modified food

- The genetic modification (GM) of food is a controversial practice as it involves altering the genetic blueprints of living organisms. Its advocates claim such products will make agriculture sustainable, eliminate world hunger, cure diseases and improve public health. But critics say GM producers are only interested in patenting their foods and seeds, and selling them for profit.
- In the US, at least 50 GM foods are already grown and sold, with dozens more under development. The fear is that these foods and crops are becoming widely dispersed into the food chain with no regard for their potential impact.
- Most supermarket-processed foods are now said to show traces of GM ingredients, and it's clearly an area in need of further independent research.

Organic foods

- The range of organic foods available is increasing all the time. Among the food types it already encompasses are fruit, vegetables, bread, meat, desserts, and beers. But with demand in the UK outstripping supply there can be shortages.
- The bigger purchasers, notably the supermarkets, overcome this by importing organic produce. It's forecast that the proportion of organic fruit and vegetable sales in supermarkets will grow to around 20 percent over the next few years. And while organic food remains dearer than conventional produce, the difference is expected to narrow.

How to buy organic

- If you want to buy organic goods, look out for the label "organic", which is a legal quality standard. Look also for products with the Soil Association logo or the phrase "Grown to UK Register of Organic Food Standards".
- Organic foods are also sold all over the UK in box schemes. These are a direct form of marketing: a producer delivers boxes containing a mixture of organic fruit and vegetables to small shops, community centres, or even to your door.
- Due to the higher cost, such schemes tend to exist only in the more affluent parts of the country.

Avoiding additives

- Food additives are widely used to preserve food. Whether they have any side effects is the subject of much debate. Not all additives are the product of modern know-how, of course. People have for centuries used salt to preserve meats and fish, added herbs and spices to improve flavours, and preserved fruit with sugar.
- Perhaps the most criticised additive is monosodium glutamate. Found in some powdered soups and instant gravies, among other foods, it's said that it can cause brain damage if consumed in large quantities. A maximum daily intake of 2 grams ($^1/_8$oz) is, therefore, recommended.
- Additive usage is strictly regulated, so there shouldn't be too much to worry about. If you do develop an allergy, try to identify the aggravating ingredient by studying the food labels.

Food supplements

Too many of us stuff ourselves with greasy fast foods and home-delivered pizzas. They fill a hole but deny the body the nutrients it needs. Food supplements can help you out.

Nutrient deficiency

- If you eat a balanced diet you'll usually get enough vitamins and minerals and taking supplements is unlikely to improve your health. But it is possible to become nutrient deficient.
- A main cause of deficiency is an increasing reliance on fast, processed, and highly-refined foods. Another is that the nutritional value of our food is only as good as the soil it's grown in. The processing, packaging, and freezing of food can also deplete it of nutrients.
- Men struggling with poverty, or drug or alcohol dependency are less likely to have an adequate diet, and certain chronic diseases also interfere with the body's ability to absorb nutrients. Long-term medication can also upset the body's metabolism. Any of these reasons may make supplements beneficial.

Choosing a supplement

- You should consult your doctor before taking nutrient supplements. For most, general multivitamin and multimineral tablets will suffice. They should contain vitamins A, B, C, D, and E as well as calcium, magnesium, potassium, iron, zinc, selenium, and copper, among other trace minerals.
- Some supplement brands contain several times the recommended daily dosage. Your body may ignore the excess, but not always – too much vitamin A, for example, can cause hair loss and skin irritation.
- Some supplements work by releasing small quantities of the ingredients over a prolonged period of time, which is particularly useful in the case of water-soluble vitamins.
- Products that promote themselves as "natural" and "organic" are of minimal benefit, and in many cases chemical solvents are used to extract the nutrients.

Natural supplements – do they work?

Evening primrose oil This flower oil contains a high amount of gamma linolenic acid that can help conditions such as eczema and rheumatoid arthritis. For eczema, experts recommend adults take four 500mg capsules a day to counter itching, and eight to twelve 500mg capsules for more severe cases.

Fish oils Fish oils, such as cod liver oil, are a rich source of vitamins A and D, which are needed for healthy skin, teeth, and gums. Fish oils are also said to help sufferers of rheumatoid arthritis, eczema, acne, and psoriasis.

Royal jelly. Royal jelly is packed with the B vitamins, vitamin C, minerals, plus amino acids and fatty acids. There is as yet no scientific evidence to back them up, but advocates of royal jelly claim it can alleviate a wide variety of health complaints including acne, allergies, anxiety, arthritis, baldness, headaches, and impotence.

Ginseng Well known as an aphrodisiac, ginseng has also been used for centuries in the East as a general medicine. Research suggests it can improve stamina and concentration, reduce stress and tiredness, and protect against radiation.

Superoxide dismutase (SOD) This enzyme is reputed to counter free radicals, which have a damaging effect on health. SOD is produced naturally in the body but supplementation can bolster the immune system. Taken via injections, it has been shown to benefit sufferers of rheumatoid arthritis, Crohn's disease, and ulcerative colitis.

Lecithin Lecithin is said to help prevent heart disease and act as a slimming aid. As a natural diuretic, lecithin can inhibit weight gain by removing excess fluid. It's an emulsifier which breaks down fat and helps absorb cholesterol into the body's cells. It's made by the liver and is found in egg yolks and soya beans.

Garlic Garlic may improve cardiovascular health by reducing blood pressure and high cholesterol levels. As an antioxidant it can also help strengthen your immunity.

(These natural substances do not ensure good health by themselves – always maintain a good, balanced diet.)

Nurturing relationships

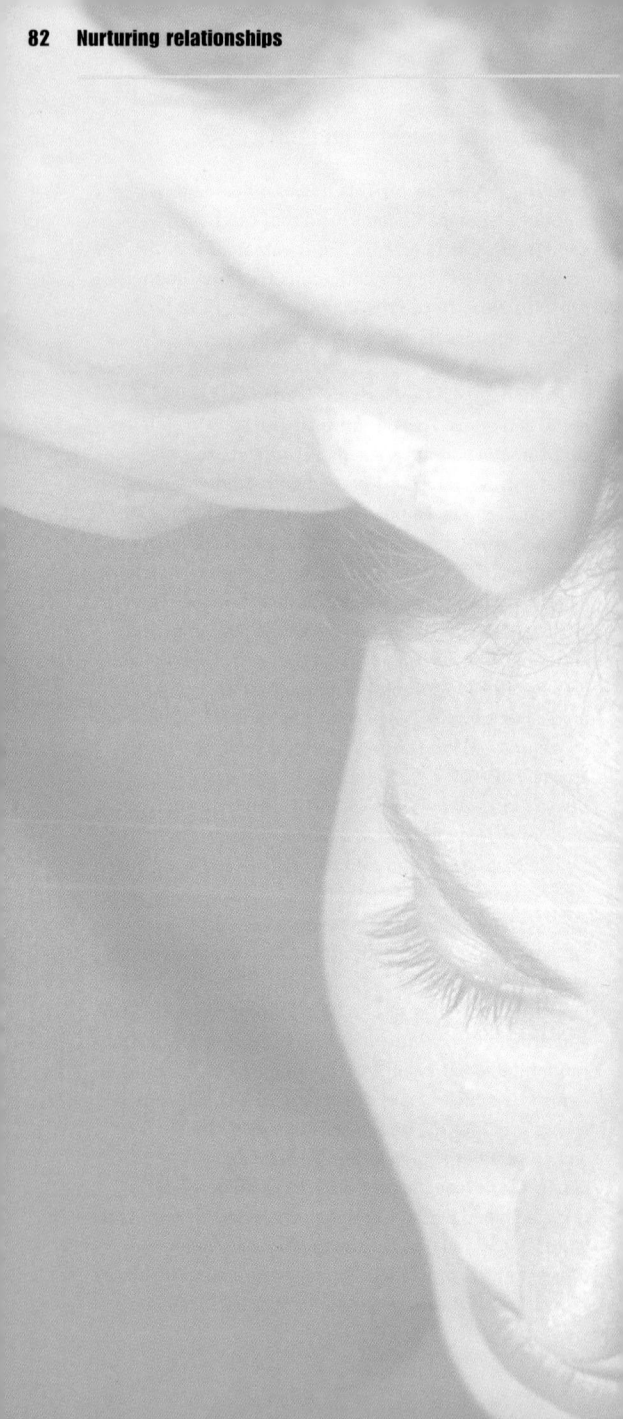

Nurturing relationships

Communicating well
Body language
The art of listening
Understand one another
Revisiting passion
Keeping love alive
Back in the market

Communicating well

Some of us are chatty, some of us are quiet. But many of us find it difficult to discuss our relationships. It's a male design fault that can be overcome.

Talk your way forward

- Talking is probably the single most important ingredient in a successful relationship. By talking about your hopes and dreams, and discussing your plans and aspirations, you and your partner will bond and lock into each other's psyches.
- Such closeness and understanding generates intimacy, making good communication also the foundation for great sex.
- Talking is not always easy. Some people are naturally more taciturn than others. And when there's a conflict between you and your partner, it can be all too easy to side-step the matter and say nothing.
- Psychologists say it's important to be able to talk openly and candidly about your relationship, including any problems that are associated with it. There may be a thin chance that by avoiding an issue, it will disappear with time. But it's far more likely to fester.
- If you don't talk openly, you may develop a relationship that seems smooth on the outside but lacks the depth of understanding required for long-term harmony.

Men are from Mars

- The great divide between the sexes in past centuries may have narrowed but differences still remain. As John Gray writes in *Men are from Mars, Women are from Venus*, "Not only do men and women communicate differently, but they think, feel, perceive, react, respond, love, need, and appreciate differently."
- Though people may disagree, the defining difference seems to be that women crave intimacy while men fear losing their independence. This, of course, is a generalisation. But most men have probably identified with it at some time.
- The articles about "what he really thinks" in women's magazines seem to underline communication differences.

Let's talk about sex

For most women, verbal interaction is a vital precursor to physical intimacy. Most women like to feel cocooned in love, trust, and warmth before moving towards sex. That's why going to bed early just to talk can be so good. Confiding your worries can be a turn-on for women. They'll regard it as a sign of strength rather than weakness. And once you're both relaxed and comfortable, physical intimacy is almost sure to follow.

Control your moods

Losing your temper is unlikely to do your relationship any good. Here are some measures to keep your temper in check:
- Are you really feeling angry or are you allowing anger to replace another emotion, such as envy or shame?
- Look at the matter from your partner's point of view.
- Pinpoint the source of your anger. Is it the issue that's just arisen or the touch-paper for a more deep-rooted problem?
- Put the problem in perspective. Tell your partner that your angry feelings do not threaten your underlying love for her.
- Don't bring up old grudges – stick to the current matter.

Top tips for cheerful chatting

1. **First steps** Just start talking. Getting any dialogue going is better than waiting for that elusive "best moment".

2. **Walkie-talkie** If you find it difficult to talk face-to-face, go for a walk together. The free atmosphere of outdoors should help free your tongue.

3. **Express yourself** Although you may find it difficult to express your feelings, you must try. Your partner is sure to appreciate the effort.

4. **Build up to it** If there's an issue you want to discuss but find difficult to voice, build up to it by talking about easier, related topics.

5. **Bed rules** Remember that bed is a place for trust. It is not the venue to make a shocking revelation to your partner.

Body language

Despite your best intentions to say the right thing, your body may already be saying something else. So learn about some of the ways your body transmits information, and don't let it betray you again.

Body language facts

- By paying more attention to eye contact, tone of voice, posture, proximity, and hand gestures, we can better assess how our words are being received.
- A person who doesn't maintain eye contact could be feeling shy, nervous, or guilty.
- Approaching someone sideways is regarded as being less confrontational than approaching head-on.
- Before you speak, a woman has probably taken in information about your posture and what mood you're in.

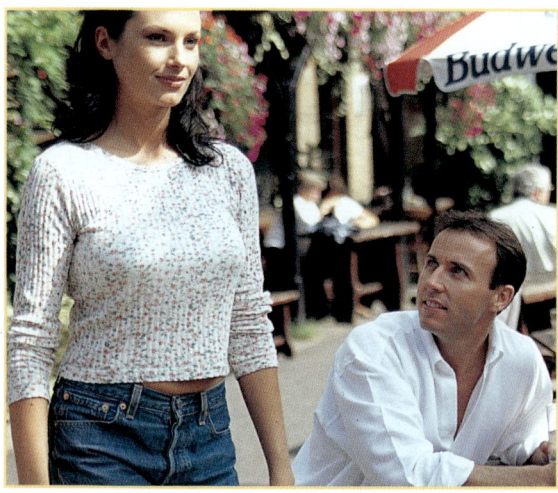

If you think body language is a load of poppycock, consider this: experts say that 58 percent of communication is made by body language, 38 percent by tone of voice, and just 7 percent by actual words.

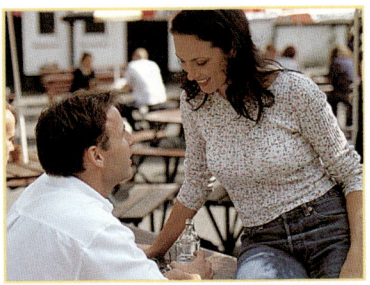

Open arms are a sure sign of receptiveness. To show we're listening we tend to bring our hand up to our cheek or chin, but if we support our head with a hand, we're obviously bored.

To show sincerity, we often show the palms of our hands. If we feel anxious our palms sweat, which may lead to hand wringing. We also make ourselves feel more secure by clasping our hands in front of our groin.

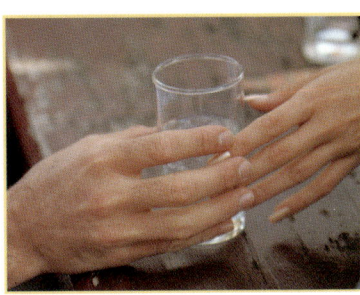

Other give-aways

NECK SCRATCHING
According to some body language specialists, when you lie there's a muscular reaction in your neck that you relieve by pulling at your collar.

FIRM HANDSHAKES
A firm handshake shows that you're unarmed and have nothing to hide. But don't let it become a power struggle.

FOLDED ARMS
Arms folded across your chest while you're making direct eye contact is a sign of a challenge or even aggression.

FLUFF INSPECTION
When we don't agree with something but feel reluctant to say so, we often exhibit some displacement activity, such as turning our face away from the speaker and picking imaginary bits of fluff from our clothes.

The art of listening

Listening to your partner can be as valuable as praising her. It shows you love, value, and respect her. It's also a tailor-made skill for those of us who are really rather lazy.

Listen up

- Listening to your partner is just as important as learning to express your feelings. You may think she could talk for her country, but that doesn't mean she doesn't want to be heard.
- Listen closely to what she's saying, or trying to say. If something has upset her, she may only allude to it as a means of sounding out whether she can fully confide in you. If you've been listening carefully, you can draw her out.
- To do this you must make an effort to hear what she's saying instead of predicting or guessing what you think she's saying. Let her talk freely about whatever she wants, however trivial it may sometimes seem to you. For her, good dialogue is pivotal to the relationship.

Paying someone to listen

- We all confide in our mates about important matters, but often not as much as our partners do in their girlfriends.
- Sometimes you can have a relationship problem that you cannot resolve between the two of you and that would be inappropriate to throw at a friend. This is when it can be worthwhile paying a professional counsellor to listen to you.
- Many men have a problem with counselling – as borne out by the fact that 90 percent of all people in therapy are women. But the benefits can be substantial.
- An experienced counsellor will listen objectively to what you both have to say. The counsellor may also ask to talk to both of you individually. You may well find the experience immediately therapeutic.
- If you find it a struggle, try to persevere. Be honest and rational. And focus on what it is you are trying to achieve – cementing your relationship. If you've got the will, a good counsellor should be able to help get you there.

Top ten tips for better listening

1. **Pay attention** The most important thing is to stay focused. Don't let your mind wander off.

2. **Get a grip** Don't just hear the words. Make sure you understand what your partner means by them.

3. **Get specific** Try to sense the feelings beyond the words as much as the words themselves. If your partner is trying to tell you something that's awkward or difficult, she may resort to vague language. Don't take these words at face value to avoid the problem. Ask her to be more specific.

4. **Avoid presumption** Don't start preparing an answer before you've fully heard what she has to say.

5. **Avoid distraction** Don't be distracted by the TV or the football scores. She will feel undervalued and will probably clam up, creating a distance between the two of you.

6. **Maintain eye contact** Show her you're paying her attention by maintaining eye contact. Nod occasionally to give encouragement.

7. **Hear her out** Resist the instinct to reply on impulse. If she's saying something critical about you, let her finish saying it. She may be right or she may be wrong. But give her the respect of a full hearing. Then you can have your say.

8. **Clarify** If you're not sure what she's saying, ask questions. She'd rather be asked to clarify a point than have you second-guess what she's saying and get it wrong.

9. **Be patient** By and large, don't interrupt her.

10. **Look out for hidden meanings** Listen for the nuances in what she's saying. This applies both when she is speaking to you alone and when you are among a group of people. There may be situations in public when she is trying to communicate something to you without anyone else noticing. Listen up.

Understand one another

Unfortunately, your partner didn't come with a service manual. So to get to know her you'll have to study and revise. Just don't assume that her needs are the same as yours.

Support your partner

- If you think you can support your partner as you do your friends, you may need to think again. A woman does not want to be left alone to overcome a problem by herself. She wants your active support. Patience and tenderness are the key.
- Give her your undivided attention and, when she feels ready, she will share her troubles with you. Don't feel redundant if her trouble is to do with something at her work over which you cannot have any influence. Just listening, hugging, and giving general support can be what she needs.

Find out more

- As you may have spotted, women can be tremendously complex. But if you want to make her happy, you've got to know everything about her – her hopes, fears, beliefs – what makes her tick. You may share common interests that brought you together in the first place, but study her in more detail.
- If you're struggling to gauge what she wants, ask her. You may get a very blunt answer but at least it will give you a clearer picture. She will appreciate the effort you've made.

Foreplay all day

- Foreplay is more than a brief fumble before having sex. For women, sexual response begins long before you get into the bedroom. Women like to feel connected to you for a much longer period of time. Little expressions of love and affection through the day go a lot further than late-night fumbling.
- If closeness is built up slowly, women find it much easier to open up sexually. So listen to her, buy her flowers, and tell she's beautiful – and mean it!

Best friends

Most women want their partner to be their best friend too. As most new relationships develop, there comes a time when you will probably supplant her closest girlfriend as her number one intimate. Sex has very little to do with it. You will achieve this best friend status by cherishing your partner and showing her every respect. Be sure to listen to your partner without judgement or impatience. By sharing the ups and downs of life, you can be best friends for life.

Getting into hot water

So much for feminism and "new man" culture. It seems that many women still covet men who have money and power over those who offer love and sensitivity. In a study conducted by David Buss, Professor of Psychology at the University of Texas, 10,000 women in 37 cultures across the world were asked what they wanted in a mate. Across all cultures, including those in the West, women universally say they desire the following attributes in the order given:

- Money and wealth
- Social status and power
- Someone older – by 3–4 years on average
- Ambition
- Dependability and intelligence
- Love and commitment

The first five traits provide a woman with the security she seeks to optimise the circumstances for raising a family. Older, more intelligent men of good social status offer all the evolutionary advantages – better housing, better food, better education, and better access to health care. Perhaps this is the driving force, as much as fear of redundancy, that impels so many men to work long hours in an attempt to climb the corporate ladder. Within this context, it can seem as though love and commitment are just lucky bonuses.

Revisiting passion

The sparks of passion glittered like a firework in the early days. Then after a while you both came back down to earth. But with a little planning you can relight the romance.

Long-term maintenance

- Most relationships are fuelled in the early stages by an intense passion. But after a while the gas can start to run out. This is normal, although it can be disappointing. It's at this point that you've got to work at the relationship.
- In the long term, you only get out of it what you put in. This means making the time to share with your partner lots of fun and laughter, sex and tenderness, dreams and adventures. You should also try to re-cultivate that romantic flair that so impressed her when you were courting.
- You may have ditched such strategies once you'd won her, but women crave romance all the time. So reacquaint yourself with the local florist shop, light some candles, and cook her a seductive dinner. It will help strengthen the bond between you.

The dating game again

You can rekindle the passion you once had by starting to date your partner again. Take her out and try travelling separately to the meeting point. Here are some dating suggestions:
- Book a table at a restaurant you know she'll like. Give her some warning of how smart it is. She'll only feel comfortable if she's suitably dressed.
- Go to a play, ballet, or a concert. Make sure it's something she will want to see, not just something you want to see.
- Take her somewhere beautiful and romantic, like a country-house hotel. The more secluded and private, the better.
- Take her dancing.
- Do something she hasn't done before. Go to the opera, book a hot-air balloon ride, or go to a health farm.
- Use your imagination. You don't have to spend a fortune – the aim is to get away from your usual surroundings.

Starting a sexual fire

For some couples, it's not a case of rekindling the flame but of lighting it in the first place. Maybe you started with the merest of sexual sparks. Don't worry as the best part of your relationship life may lie ahead. Studies show that those having the most emotionally and physically fulfilling sex lives are in long-term relationships, and for many the best sex comes later in life.

Relighting a fire

A few simple touches may reinvigorate your relationship:
- **Flowers** Buy her some – all women love them
- **Say it** Tell her you love her – face-to-face, by 'phone, fax, letter, email – it doesn't matter
- **Surprise** Take her out somewhere you know she likes on the spur of the moment
- **Remember** Birthdays, Valentine's day, and anniversaries are important to her
- **Gifts** Be it pricey perfume or cheap chocolates, make sure it's something she likes, not just something you like
- **Cook** Show her that you can rustle up a romantic meal without using a tin-opener
- **Sex** Reignite those sexual fires with some adventurous sex

Top tips for keeping sex alive

1. **Don't just have sex in bed** Get out of the bedroom. Try the settee, the floor, the bath, or the kitchen table. For extra adventure, get out into the garden or into the back of the car.
2. **Act out a fantasy** Pretend you're both single and go separately to a bar or club. Chat her up and take her to a hotel for the night.
3. **Dressing up** If she's prepared to, ask her to dress up and act as though she's visiting you in a hotel room.
4. **Buy sex aids** There are plenty of sex toys and other accessories to pep up the action. But make sure she's comfortable with what you're proposing.
5. **Three's a crowd** Suggesting a threesome is not to be recommended. Sex is a very emotional act, especially for her. Introducing a third person more often than not has a damaging long-term impact on a relationship.

Keeping love alive

Love, like a weedy pot plant, can take an awful lot of nurturing to maintain. It can be hard work, but the rewards repay the effort.

What's in it for you?

- Establishing a happy relationship can be hard work – but it's worth it. Despite macho qualms about losing independence, men need a good relationship as much as women.
- Studies show that happily married men enjoy a healthier and longer life than their single counterparts. They also suffer less illness. Why this is the case isn't certain, but a happy home life with a loving partner, good food, good sex, and emotional fulfilment probably play a part.

The "c" word

- Relationship problems and conflicts arise, and the need to compromise your own desires for the sake of your partner's can prove challenging. It's all too easy to want to graze on greener grass, but the novelty of a new partner can soon wear off, leaving you feeling empty and degraded.
- A more rewarding response is to show some of the dreaded "c" – commitment. Commitment means you can surmount any problem that threatens to separate you and your partner.

Dealing with conflict

Even the strongest relationships experience conflicts, but there are strategies to limit their impact. Regard a conflict as an abstract third-party interloper that both you and your partner need to fight off together. Remember that your aim is not to win an argument but to restore love and harmony to the relationship. This is a good time to practise your communication skills – many men tend to avoid conflict by retreating out of the room, but it will not solve problems with your partner.

Top tips for love and peace

1. **Compatibility** For long-term relationships, compatibility is essential. This means more than sharing similar values and political views. It means existing on a similar wavelength – one that also accepts you both have your differences.

2. **Communication** Face-to-face communication every day is regarded as a fundamental building block for a sturdy relationship. Only by talking properly and very regularly can two individuals expect their lives to converge.

3. **Sex** Some couples can exist happily without sex, but they are few and far between. A warm, loving sex life is almost a prerequisite for a strong relationship.

4. **Individuality** However close you become, you'll always remain separate entities. Respect your partner's interests and allow her time to pursue her hobbies. It's unhealthy to spend every minute of every day with one another.

5. **Compromise** A good relationship undeniably dilutes each person's individual identity. You'll probably have to compromise some of your interests for the good of the relationship. This is not the same as being under her thumb. The skill is to compromise graciously without resentment.

6. **Honesty** Being honest with your partner is crucial. And being found out for being dishonest about something important will seriously jeopardise your relationship.

7. **Forgiveness** The person who forgives will not be forgotten. If your partner has stepped out of line and regrets it, she will love you all the more if you can find it in you to forgive her.

8. **Investment** You've got to invest in the relationship. Giving, caring, and sharing are key ingredients for a happy team. Those who invest for longer are likely to end up richer.

9. **Time** Today's high-pressure lifestyles and the demands of a family can put time at a premium, but you must spend quality time together to have a happy relationship.

Back in the market

Breaking up can be painful or liberating, or both. But now you're single again there's a mass of women waiting to meet you. So shape up and get out there.

Fools rush in

- Finding yourself single after a long relationship can be very tough. As well as the emotional impact, you have to come to terms with your new single social status.
- It depends why the split occurred, of course, but unless you have a heart of stone, your emotional foundations may be disturbed. You may feel vulnerable and the danger is that you'll leap at the first half-likely woman you meet. This may be unfair on both of you. Try to broaden your horizons and take your time to re-find your feet – and have some fun.

Address your needs

- At this point you need to define what you're looking for from the opposite sex. You may feel ready to revel in your new-found freedom, in which case you may be up for casual sex with any woman who takes your eye. But if you're looking for a new long-term partner, you'll be using different criteria.
- Avoid comparing women to your ex – this is unlikely to be helpful. Everyone's unique, so judge each accordingly. What you're looking for is your female complement. It may take time to find her, but she's out there.

Time to tidy up

This might be a good time to take a look at your physical self. Did you let yourself go a bit in your previous relationship? You're back in business now, so maybe you could do with losing some weight and firming up those muscles. Exercise will help increase self-confidence. And what about your clothes? Would a new shirt or jacket boost your pulling power? While you're at it, tidy up your flat or house. Clean surroundings will also boost your mood.

Top places to meet and date

If chatting a stranger up in a pub, bar, or club is not your style, try some of these options:

- Friends. Use your friends' social and business circles to meet new people.
- Parties. House parties are always a good bet.
- Work. About 10 percent of couples meet at work, so join your company's social or sports club.
- Classes. Adult education and evening classes are a good bet.
- Dance lessons. This is an excellent option as women almost always outnumber men.
- Clubs and societies. Many local clubs organise events, such as dances, hikes, barbecues, bike rides, lectures, and film nights.
- Political or community action groups. Do your bit for the locality at the same time.
- Dating agencies. Introduction agencies no longer carry a stigma.
- Gyms. Many gym-goers are really taking an opportunity to display themselves.

She's agreed to go out with you and the pressure's on to take her somewhere other than your local pub, try:

- Unusual or romantic restaurants. High-street pizza outlets and fast food shops don't have the same effect.
- Outdoor activities. Go walking in the country or by the river.
- Cultural interests. Visit an art gallery or museum.
- Driving. Go for a motor in the country.
- Book readings. Many bigger bookshops host readings by authors.
- Wine-tasting. Some wine shops hold wine-tasting evenings.
- Concerts, plays, or operas. Take her to see the performances that everyone's talking and writing about.
- Bizarre events. Take her where she doesn't usually go, such as to greyhound-racing, bingo, or a casino.
- Desperate measures. If all else fails, invite her round to watch a romantic foreign-language film.

98 First impressions

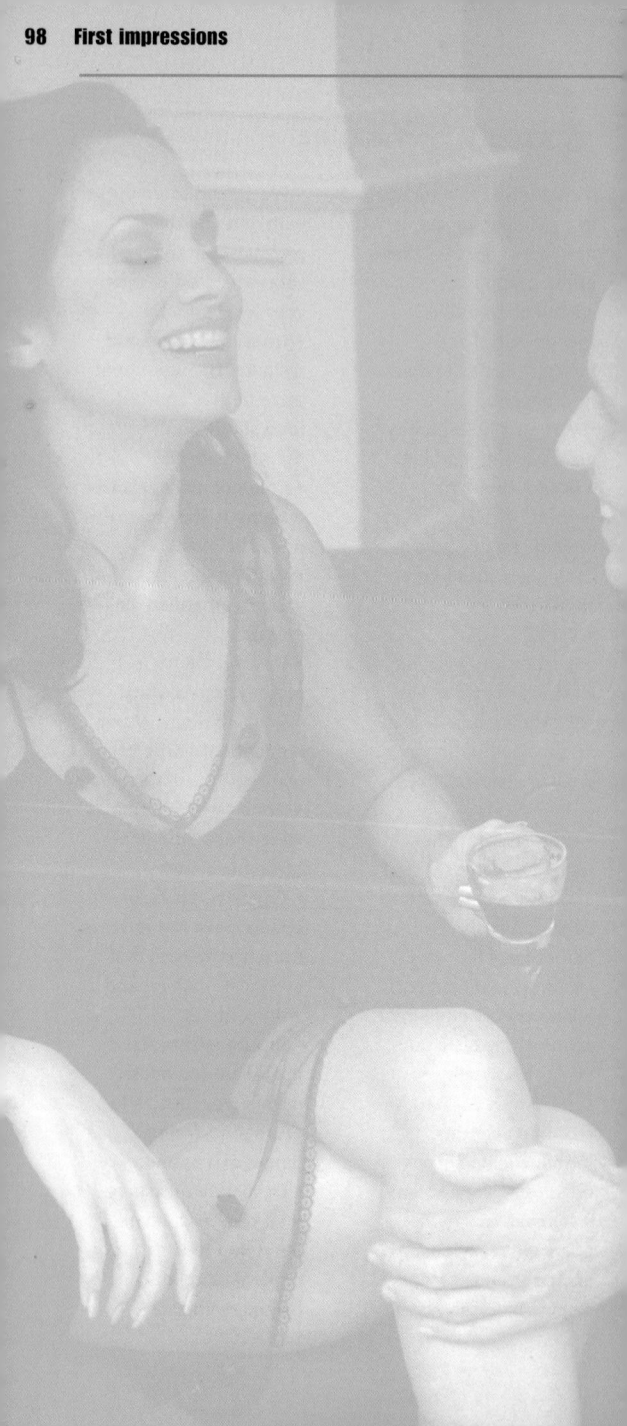

First impressions

First moves
Dressing with sense
Suits you sir
First base to home run

First moves

Chatting up a stranger can be difficult. There's a fine line between flirting and being a nuisance. But like chess, a good opening gambit could allow you to enjoy the end-game.

How confident are you?

- Approaching someone you fancy can reduce many a man to a quivering wreck. Of course, it all depends on where you are. If you're at a party or in a nightclub, the unwritten rules of social interaction are in your favour.
- Don't assume every woman at the bar wants to be chatted up. But if you do take a shine to a complete stranger, try to make eye contact. If she holds your look for a moment more than necessary, don't assume she must be short-sighted. She may like what she sees. You could then offer to buy her a drink.

Gaining confidence

- Having made contact you need to reassure her that you're not a complete nutter. Don't invade her personal space. Ask open questions and listen carefully to what she says.
- The best approach may be to regard her initially as a potential new friend rather than a girlfriend. This should limit any likelihood of becoming tongue-tied. You can then attempt to gain her confidence by telling her who you are and what you do. If you get this far, it should be her turn to buy you a drink.

The right impression

- If you're looking for a one-night stand then pretending you're all set to be a film star might be worthwhile. But if you're earmarking her as a potential girlfriend, honesty is best.
- Admitting you're a poorly-paid office clerk may not sweep her off her feet, but it should get you marked as honest. Still, probably best not to say how lowly-paid at this stage.
- She may try to gauge how much emotional baggage you have. If you're still traumatised by your ex's decision to join a nunnery, keep quiet for now and aim to swap 'phone numbers.

Top ten tips for a good chat-up

1. **Just good friends** Regard a woman you meet for the first time as a potential friend rather than a partner. This should make it easier to start a conversation if you're nervous.

2. **Ask open questions** Ask ones that require more than a yes or no answer. For example, ask her why she thought a film was good or how she got her current job.

3. **Be original** Whenever possible, approach your target with a comment that's just for her, such as "That's a beautiful bracelet" or "What do you think of that book?".

4. **Keep it simple** Say something like "What's the pasta like here?", or "Is that a good wine you're drinking?".

5. **Keep it upbeat** Most women prefer men with enthusiasm, energy, and wit. Harping on about how slow the bar staff are or your struggles to get a taxi are negative and boring.

6. **Offer to help** It's possible to open a door for a woman or offer to carry a heavy bag for her without being patronising.

7. **Say something funny** Women love men who can make them laugh. But be careful. A witty off-the-cuff remark is what you're looking for, not a decrepit old "knock, knock" joke or that sexist gag you heard down the pub.

8. **Avoid corny chat-up lines** Unless you have the ability to imbue a clichéd chat-up line with enough irony to show you don't mean it, forget it. And anyway, she's probably heard them all before.

9. **Listen carefully** Attentive listening is an under-rated skill and one that will make her feel respected. Respond to what she says – don't just plough on with what you were going to say anyway.

10. **Compliment her** Everyone likes to be told how good they're looking. With a little skill you can say this without it sounding embarrassing.

Dressing with sense

Fashions come and go, but some clothes remain impervious to such whims. Add your own touches to the basics and you too can be in vogue.

The basics

No matter what you have to wear at work, every professional man's wardrobe should contain a few basic items. You can then buy other clothes to create your own image. Items that can be mixed and matched will prove the most flexible:
- A dark suit. This could be navy blue, grey, charcoal, or pinstripe. By dressing it up or down with different coloured shirts and ties, it should be suitable for most formal occasions, such as interviews, weddings, and funerals.
- A navy blazer, for a casual-smart look
- A white cotton shirt
- A blue cotton shirt
- Two ties, preferably silk or cotton. Avoid comedy ties unless you want to look like a yuppie in a 1980s time warp.
- A pair of khaki trousers
- A pair of blue or black jeans

Colour matters

The colour of your clothes should match and also complement your complexion. It's an inaccurate science but some colour combinations will make you look fit and well, while others will make you seem pale and tired. Here are some dos and don'ts for various skin types:
- **Blond or fair** Wear lighter-coloured clothes, such as salmon, ivory, and light grey. Bold ties work well against soft colours.
- **Brown** Wear neutral, basic, and bold colours – not deep tones.
- **Olive** Stick to natural colours and avoid olive drab or army khaki. Offset this with some colour in your tie or shirt.
- **Black** Avoid light pastels, greys, and navys, which can look drab. Stick to bold colours, black, and softer blues.
- **Ruddy** A good combination is navy blue with a red tie and khaki trousers. Try to create a contrast in your clothes.
- **Yellow** Avoid black and choose neutrals, khakis, and greens.

Top ten tips for buying clothes

1. **Second opinions** If you lack confidence buying clothes, persuade your partner or a friend to shop with you. Listen to their advice but don't feel compelled by it.

2. **Value for money** Spend as much as you can on suits and jackets. These items are good investments. A cheap jacket will always look cheap no matter how fashion changes.

3. **Don't buy too much at once** The danger is you won't think clearly about what will match other clothes in your wardrobe.

4. **Always try clothes on** Use a shop's changing rooms. Manufacturing processes vary and not all clothes that show your size on the label will necessarily fit you well.

5. **Don't be impatient** If you've tried on several pairs of trousers and none of them feels quite right, don't buy any of them. You've probably already got items at the back of your wardrobe that aren't quite right.

6. **Leave enough room** Jackets and blazers should not be so tight that they strain across the chest.

7. **Standing and sitting** When trying on trousers, make sure they feel comfortable when walking and when seated. If possible, try them on with the shoes you'd wear them with.

8. **Shoe fitting** When trying on shoes, beware that feet swell in hot weather and when you walk long distances. Walk around the shop to gauge the comfort of the shoes and wear socks of appropriate thickness.

9. **Go natural** Although today's synthetic materials are vastly improved, look for fabrics that contain no less than 80 percent natural fibres. Many blended fabrics with up to 20 percent synthetic materials provide style, quality, and easy maintenance.

10. **What socks** Pure cotton socks allow your feet to breathe better than any other fabric.

Suits you sir

What looks good on you should dictate what you wear, not the latest fashion. Some types of clothing may be trendy but if they don't suit your size or shape, don't wear them.

Style for all

You can minimise mistakes by following a few general principles. Slim men should consider double-breasted suits because they give an impression of bulk. Heavier men are more flattered by single-breasted suits. Pleated trousers are good for all body shapes as they are slimming – tight cuts can be fine if you're on the slim side but not if you've got tree trunks for thighs.

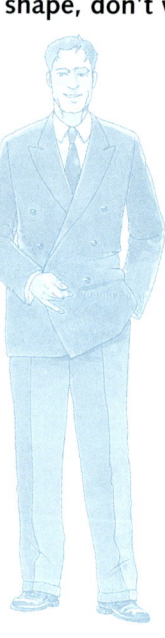

Tall and slim

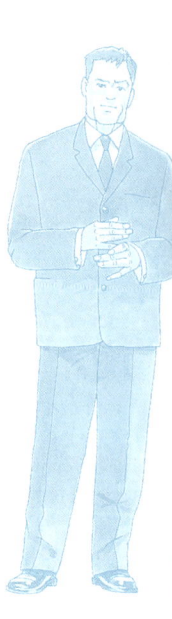

Short medium-heavy

	Tall and slim	Short medium-heavy
Suit styles Styles to flatter height and build	Single- or double-breasted to flatter the perfect figure	Single-breasted adds height and slenderises
Shirt styles Flattering fits and smart finishes	European cuts or basic fits display a slender waist	Looser basic fits distract the eye from thicker waists
Trouser styles Pleated, regular, tight, or loose styles	Pleated, tight, or regular cuts – with turn-ups if skinny	Pleated or regular cuts create an illusion of height

Choosing a shirt

Shirt styles can be chosen from four main fits. A basic fit is loose at the waist. The athletic fit is wide across the shoulders and narrow at the waist. The loose fit is oversize and full through the body, and the European cut is a tapered dress shirt style.

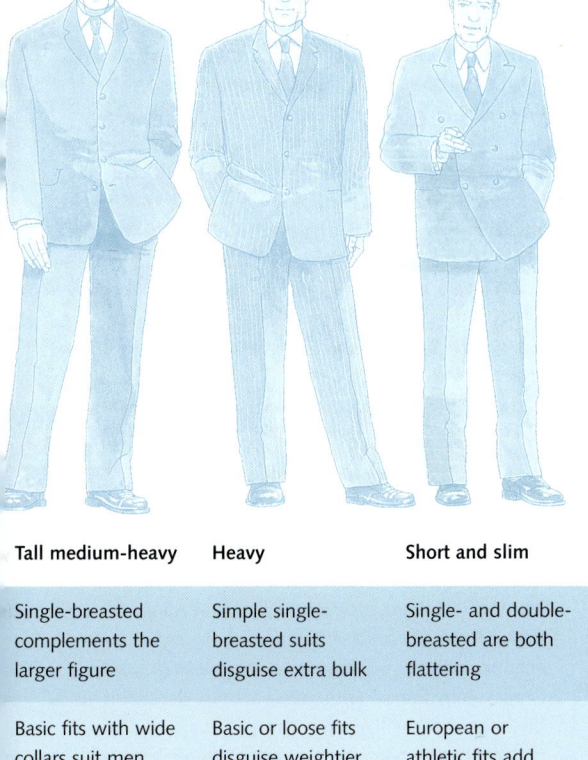

Tall medium-heavy	Heavy	Short and slim
Single-breasted complements the larger figure	Simple single-breasted suits disguise extra bulk	Single- and double-breasted are both flattering
Basic fits with wide collars suit men with thick necks	Basic or loose fits disguise weightier physiques	European or athletic fits add fullness to the body
Pleated or regular cuts with tailored trousers flatter	Pleated or loose, with a pinstripe to disguise heavy legs	Pleated, tight, or regular cut straight trousers add height

First base to home run

Starting a relationship is one of life's great experiences. But it's also a time of uncertainty as passions can run high.

Consolidating your gains

- You've started seeing someone and now you face a dilemma. If the first couple of meetings went well, you could be on the brink of starting a full relationship, with all the emotional pitfalls that entails. It can be a big step.
- If you want to develop the relationship further, one way to show your new partner how much she means to you is to introduce her to your friends. This carries significance as it shows her that you're willing to make a public statement.
- How she handles meeting your friends can also be an indication of her feelings for you. If she likes you, she will want to make a good impression and may be a little nervous. Reassure her that you wouldn't introduce her to your best friends if you didn't think a lot of her. And if you really want to stress your feelings for her, you could take that critical extra step and ask her if she'd like to meet your parents.

Love or lust?

A new relationship can be a time of uncertainty. While a flurry of dates can elate the spirits, a corner of your mind will be wondering where it's all heading. Are you falling in love or lust? Who's setting the pace? You will need to analyse your emotions. Do you think you're being totally honest with her or are you deceiving her in the hope that she'll sleep with you? Analysing her motives can be hard when you don't know her very well. The best policy is to take things slowly. If you're both falling in love, then you'll both be prepared to be patient before having sex. The problem is when one partner has a different expectation from the other. If one of you is being dishonest, the other is sure to get hurt.

What men really want

- There is a widely held view that men need sex more than women. This is not true. Many women say their sexual drive is as strong or stronger than their partner's. There does, however, seem to be some truth in the perception that men are more interested in casual sex. Women, on the other hand, place more emphasis on the need for an emotional connection before having sex.
- Men seem more able to separate the physical act from any feelings of love. This difference – albeit a generalisation – between the genders is borne out by society's primitive double standard: men who sleep around are "studs", whereas women who do the same are "slags".
- When you're starting a relationship, be careful not to be sexually aggressive, but gauge your partner's feelings carefully. She may be just as keen as you to have a roll in the hay, but she probably wants to feel emotionally secure first.
- When she says she's ready it means she trusts you and, hopefully, she's right. Sex creates an emotional bond, so be sure of what you really, really want before you get undressed.

In the aftermath

- How you behave after sex will be taken by your partner as an indication of how you feel for her. If you subscribe to the "wham, bam, thank you mam" school of post-coital interaction, she's unlikely to be impressed. Most women want to be cuddled and cherished after intercourse. This is also a better time to tell her you love her than during sex.
- Unfortunately, men often feel naturally tired after having sex and are prone to falling asleep. Try to resist this, for a while at least. Snoring within a couple of minutes of great intimacy is unlikely to endear you to your new beloved.
- Giving an appraisal of how the sexual encounter went is fine if it was good. But if it was not so good, don't say so in the immediate aftermath. No one wants to be told they're a lousy lover straight away. If there was a problem you want to mention, it's far better to wait until sometime later or the next day. When you do make a comment, make it sound constructive rather than critical. We can all feel vulnerable in bed, so treat your partner as you'd like her to treat you.

Great sex

Puberty
Masturbation
Losing it
Sexual psychology
Foreplay
Massage
Sensual massage
Oral sex
Sexual phases
Male orgasms
Female orgasms
Moving the earth
Multiple orgasms
Alternatives to intercourse
Games and fantasies
Sexual aids
Dressing for sex
Potency
Aphrodisiacs
Dealing with impotency
Contraceptive methods
Sexual health

Puberty

From about the age of 10, a surge in sex hormones propels the body towards sexual maturity. The genitals develop and the body gears up to become capable of sex.

What happens exactly?

- Puberty usually starts between the ages of 10 and 15. The brain releases chemical messengers that produce sex hormones, the most important of which is testosterone.
- Testosterone prompts the testicles to grow and the scrotum to hang lower and become more wrinkled and darker. The penis becomes longer and increases in width. Pubic hair starts to grow around the penis, followed by hair growth in the armpits and on the face and chest.
- Testosterone also causes the prostrate gland and the larynx to enlarge. The latter causes the voice to become deeper. The shoulders and chest become broader and the muscles develop.

Coping with hang-ups

- Puberty is a period of great uncertainty as the body transforms itself from that of a child into that of an adult. It's very common to worry about whether you're developing too fast or too slowly, but everyone develops at a different rate. By about the age of 18, everybody reaches their natural body size.
- About 40 percent of boys experience an increase in size of one or both of their "breasts" during puberty. This can cause anxiety but, in most cases, swelling disappears within a year.

First encounters

- The blossoming of the body is matched by an increasing desire to test out its sexuality. Older teenagers feel a growing desire for physical contact, including heavy petting.
- This can be a difficult time for both sexes. Boys are fuelled both by a desire for physical gratification and peer pressure, while girls tend to be more reluctant. The result is that most boys' first fumbling experiences are awkward and disappointing.

Post-pubescent facts

- The penis has two functions: to discharge urine and to conduct semen during ejaculation. Urine and semen are carried along the penis by a tube called the urethra.
- Three muscles in the penis enable it to become erect. Two of the muscles pull the penis into its erect position, allowing blood to engorge the shaft's spongy tissue. The third muscle, at the base of the penis, contracts during ejaculation to propel semen from the testicles.
- The penis changes colour during erection, becoming darker, often with blue veins standing out on its surface.
- Most erect penises are slightly curved.
- The head of the penis, the glans, is covered in sensory nerve endings, making it one of the most erogenous parts of the body.
- The foreskin, the loose skin that covers the glans, retracts during erection to expose the penis head.
- The foreskin produces a colourless, oily substance called smegma which, if not washed, can become white and smelly. Regular, gentle washing with warm water will stop the foreskin becoming smelly or infected.
- The average penis is 6.5–10.5cm (2^1/$_2$–4in) long when flaccid and 15–18cm (6–7in) long when erect. The size and angle of erection can be affected by alcohol and tiredness, among other things.
- Despite popular belief, penis size has no correlation to body size or the size of hands, nose, or feet.
- The two male sex glands, the testicles, are contained in the scrotum, which hangs behind the penis.
- The testicles usually differ in size. The left one also normally hangs lower than the right one.
- During sexual arousal, the skin of the scrotum tightens to pull the testicles up closer to the body.
- The testicles produce sperm and also the male sex hormone, testosterone.
- Sperm takes about 3 months to fully develop.
- Sperm is first produced in puberty and production continues throughout a man's life.
- On average, each testicle produces about 1500 sperm per second.

Masturbation

It's had a bad press in the past but now views have changed – masturbation is good for you. It's cheap, it's easy, and it's fun. And best of all, you don't have to buy it flowers.

Masturbation is good

- Masturbation is still not widely discussed but it's now accepted as natural and healthy. Regular masturbation keeps sperm supply healthy by generating fresh production.
- More significantly, men can learn about their own sexual response. If you don't know how your body works when aroused, how can you expect a woman to know?
- By learning how to postpone ejaculation through masturbation you can also become a better lover.

Casting off guilt

The days when pleasuring yourself was regarded as self-abuse are long gone. Sex therapists now advocate the merits of masturbation. Tales about it causing blindness, for example, are fiction; the only harm might be misguided feelings of guilt.

Masturbation facts

- Most men masturbate regularly. Surveys reveal that 13 percent of men do it more than three times a week, 25 percent do it one to three times a week, and 15 percent do it two or three times a month.
- The Catholic church regards masturbation as sinful, and Orthodox Jews are taught never to touch their penises.
- Masturbation is good for men in older age who may be without a partner. By gaining an erection through masturbation, they can allay fears about impotency.
- Men who are not sexually active and who don't masturbate will eventually have a "wet dream", when semen is emitted during sleep.

Top ten tips for self pleasure

1. **Lubricate** Use some form of lubrication, such as baby oil or saliva, to reduce friction and increase sensation.

2. **Caress the whole genital area** Fondle your testicles and stroke the perineum – that highly sensitive strip of skin between the scrotum and anus.

3. **Use sexual fantasy** Let your imagination run riot with an imaginary situation that might well horrify you in reality.

4. **Watch a film** As people making love in the film become aroused, stimulate your penis to match the intensity of what you're watching – or read an erotic story or novel.

5. **Don't feel guilty** Masturbation is a healthy and normal activity – widely practised by men and women, both with and without partners. Indeed, surveys have found that many married men continue to masturbate on a regular basis.

6. **Take your time** You're not trying to emulate adolescent schoolboys in trying to be the first to ejaculate. The longer you take, the more powerful your climax will be.

7. **Practise self-control** Limit the pressure you use to stroke your penis and build up gradually. By learning to pace yourself you're less likely to prematurely ejaculate.

8. **Find alternatives** Seek out other ways of stimulating your penis, such as against a pillow or mattress. But be careful not to make your penis sore through friction.

9. **Vary the circumstances** Just like sex, try masturbating in different positions and in different places, such as in the bath or shower.

10. **Masturbate with a partner** Mutual masturbation is a great alternative to penetrative sex. You can either stimulate each other in turns or simultaneously. Masturbating in front of your partner is also a good way to show her how you like to be touched.

Losing it

Your virginity can either be a millstone around your neck or your most treasured possession. But when you finally do have sex for the first time, it's sure to be a tumultuous experience.

Fear of the unknown

- Choosing when to have sex for the first time is one of the most important decisions you can make. Almost everyone feels a combination of excitement and fear at the prospect.
- For many teenage boys, natural desires are compounded by peer pressure. There can also be fears about not doing it right, of climaxing too quickly, or of not being able to gain an erection.
- There can also be broader worries, such as whether to lose your virginity to a stranger at a party or to a steady girlfriend – not to mention what form of contraception to use.

It's never too late

- Delaying having sex for the first time is a good idea. Surveys show that many teenagers who lost their virginity at a young age wish they'd waited. The first time, especially for younger teenagers, is typically messy, awkward, and embarrassing.
- Those who defer intercourse until they are grown up and in a steady relationship are also more likely to be emotionally mature enough to handle the intimacy of sexual bonding.
- This is hard if your adolescent peers are egging you on to "do it". But no one should be put under pressure to have sex. The decision of when to do so is up to you alone, and when you do decide, you'll discover one of life's greatest pleasures.

Double standards

While boys are chomping at the bit to lose their virginity, young women may be struggling to live up to society's demands that they remain chaste. Despite this, by the age of 18 more than half of all young men and women have had sex. But while many boys exaggerate their sexual experience to boost their reputation, girls may well play down theirs.

Top ten tips for the first time

1. **Withstand pressure** Don't have sex for the first time before you want to. For teenage boys in particular, there's a world of difference between wanting to explore your sexuality and actually having intercourse with all its emotional implications.

2. **Don't be a pest** Peer pressure can be intense. But don't allow your mates' jibes to turn you into a pestering nuisance. Girls do not want to be pressured into having sex.

3. **Hold on** Wait until you are in a stable relationship or married. Losing your cherry to someone you really love will make the event something to cherish for the rest of your life.

4. **Plan ahead** Decide when and where you lose your virginity carefully. Choose a venue where you will have peace and privacy, well away from parents, brothers, and sisters.

5. **Practise** The first time is likely to be bewildering and possibly disappointing. Good sex is like learning to ride a bike: it takes practise, but before long the stabilisers will be off.

6. **Relax** Don't worry that you won't know what to do. And banish that common fear that you won't be able to find the vagina – just do what comes naturally.

7. **Sex is messy** As well as your own ejaculate, the vagina becomes wet with lubrication and both of you may sweat.

8. **Female virgins** If your partner is also losing her virginity, be aware that she may feel some discomfort. The hymen is a thin membrane that surrounds the entrance to the vagina at birth. It may have already been torn, but if not, it may tear when she first has sex, causing slight pain and bleeding.

9. **Contraception** It's absolutely essential and, ideally, you and your partner should discuss what contraception you will use (see p.156–163).

10. **Consider the law** Remember, in the UK sexual intercourse for heterosexuals under the age of 16 is illegal.

Sexual psychology

How can you understand your partner when you barely know yourself? Learning what has shaped you and why you react in certain ways is the first step to a healthy relationship.

The wider context

- For most people, sex is sanctioned most fully within marriage, and marriage remains a goal of most young people.
- The average age at marriage, however, has risen and more single people in their twenties and thirties are opting to be alone.
- It seems clear that the rise in social freedom has not made the attainment of emotional fulfilment any easier.

The sexual divide

- Man and woman have had an ambivalent relationship since time began: the desire for a mate often offset by confusion and bewilderment at what makes the other sex tick.
- Sociologists suggest that modern society has so rapidly blurred former distinctions (men as hunters, women as homemakers) that the human psyche has yet to fully adjust.
- Relationships founder because neither side realises that they're approaching a problem from incompatible perspectives. If you reach an impasse, there are professionals who can help.

Sex therapists

- A relationship problem may be overcome by talking to a marriage or relationship guidance counsellor.
- Problems that are psychosexual may best be dealt with by a sex therapist.
- The first step recommended by sex therapists for problems, such as impotence, is to talk to your partner.
- Sex therapists strive to make people lose their inhibitions. They also stress the importance of emotional bonding and tell couples not to be performance-driven in bed.

What the experts say

The study of human sexual behaviour has come a long way since the days when the beliefs and findings of sexologists were routinely condemned by religious and moral leaders. Modern surveys have provided important information about sexual habits and behaviour.

- **Freud.** The Austrian psychoanalyst Sigmund Freud advocated that all children had a natural desire to marry their parent of the opposite sex. He also suggested that women who had clitoral orgasms were psychologically immature compared to women who experienced vaginal ones. This aside, he helped establish a trend of clinical investigation into a previously taboo subject area.
- **Kinsey.** Alfred Kinsey was an American zoology professor who, in 1948, published a report called "Sexual Behaviour in the Human Male". It created a furore by highlighting the prevalence of masturbation, premarital sex, and extramarital affairs. His work was condemned by moralists leaders, but it did much to prompt later research into sexology.
- **Masters and Johnson.** In the late 1950s and early 1960s, two American sex researchers made a ground-breaking survey of human sexual behaviour. William Masters and Virginia Johnson observed 700 men and women conduct more than 10,000 acts of intercourse and masturbation. The book they published in 1966, *Human Sexual Response*, described in vivid physical detail what happens when men and women have sex. They concluded that sexual intercourse involved four phases: excitement, plateau, orgasm and resolution (*see p.130–131*). They also stated that women's orgasms achieved by masturbation of the clitoris were generally more intense than orgasms gained through intercourse.
- **Hite.** Shere Hite made a survey of 2000 American women in the 1970s. She reported that about 30 percent of women never achieved orgasm through intercourse, but that 95 percent could do so by masturbating. The Hite report was criticised for not being sufficiently representative of the population and for drawing subjective feminist conclusions.

Foreplay

Good sex isn't just about intercourse – it's a total sensual experience. And for women, in particular, it requires a lot of tender foreplay. Give her the time and she'll give you her all.

Prolong the enjoyment

- Many men seem to think foreplay simply delays getting down to the real business of having sex. This response denies them and their partners of a lot of pleasure.
- Foreplay is immensely enjoyable – tender kissing, cuddling, and stroking are wonderfully erotic. It helps you both relax, it generates trust, and it prepares your bodies for sex.
- While your penis become erect, the woman's vagina lengthens and produces lubrication to make penetration easier.
- By prolonging sexual contact, the body's senses move into a higher gear, enhancing the intensity of intercourse. For many men, the longer the foreplay, the stronger the orgasm.

Take it in turns

- There are times when passion and lust run high and you both want immediate, rampant sex. But there are other times when you may want to get straight down to it, while your partner wants lots of foreplay. The answer may be to take it in turns.
- Perhaps you can agree that on some occasions she will allow you to have sex before she's fully turned-on, while on other occasions you promise to provide extended foreplay.

The importance of touch

- Good foreplay requires skilled touching and caressing. Knowing how and where to touch your partner is fundamental to getting her in the mood. The skill is to tenderly caress her body using a variety of light and heavier strokes and to be aware of her responses.
- Arousing parts of your partner's body other than her breasts and genitals will give her the broadest range of sensation. Ask her to tell you what she likes best.

The three t's

Men's tendency to rush towards penetration is at odds with the three t's that women desire:

1 **Time** A woman likes a slow build-up to intercourse. Her body is a bit like a fire – it can take some time to get going but then it's red hot. So allow plenty of time for foreplay. And don't rush it – she will sense if you're becoming impatient. Engage in lots of foreplay activities until you both feel you can't wait for penetration any longer.

2 **Touch** Her whole body is an erogenous zone. With the right touches you can give her a lot of pleasure. And don't just touch – try kissing, nibbling, stroking, licking, and caressing.

3 **Talk** Verbal communication is generally more important to women than to men. To get her in the mood you should flirt with her verbally over a long period before you get undressed. Women like to feel emotionally connected, and that connection comes as much through talking as touching.

What turns them on

- **Lots of foreplay** As women generally take longer to become sexually aroused, foreplay helps your partner – and you – to become relaxed in the bedroom. The more relaxed she is, the better the sex.
- **Mood and atmosphere** Few women are unaffected by romantic and sensual environments. Good smells, sounds, and lighting go a long way to firing her up.
- **Taking the lead** Most women like to take the lead now and again and to be demonstrative in bed.
- **Feeling connected** While you may be able to focus on sex in isolation, women are generally more concerned with the entire relationship. Bad vibes are a definite turn-off. If there's friction between you, she's much less likely to be able to ignore it for sex.
- Her sexual feelings are also more generalised than yours, with less focus on the genitals.

Foreplay all day

For foreplay, think all day. Getting your partner in the mood needn't begin with the first touch. Call her at work and seduce her over the 'phone – but make sure she knows it's you.

Dirty 'phone calls

- The build-up to a night of passion can begin long before you and your partner are even in the same place. Of course, having sex isn't something that should always be planned, but you may want an evening of intimacy to look forward to.
- On such occasions you should regard foreplay as something to start during the day. Call your partner at work and tell her how much you love her and how much you are looking forward to the evening.
- If you don't mind risking giggles from your colleagues, you could be more raunchy. Ring your partner and ask her what underwear she's wearing. Or tell her how horny you're feeling.
- You know whether it's best to be suggestive or explicit. Hint at what you plan to do with her. Why not have a bouquet of flowers delivered to her at work?
- This should pep up her day and kick-start her mood well before she even gets home.

Setting the scene

- It takes more than a 'phone call to set up a romantic evening. So like a good cub scout, be prepared.
- Creating the most conducive conditions in your home is essential. This means doing the obvious things like tidying up and putting clean sheets on the bed. But it also means creating the right mood.
- Turn off that bright overhead light and turn on some dimmer lamps. Better still, light a few candles. And don't forget that most under-rated of the senses, smell. Heating essential oils can be wonderfully seductive. Some oils are merely relaxing, while others, such as lavender, jasmine, juniper, and patchouli, are known for their aphrodisiac properties.
- A little background music helps, though bear in mind that your favourite speed garage track may not be the best option. And finally, if possible, switch off your 'phone. This is not the time to be disturbed.

The delights of anticipation

- Foreplay can be both explicit and subtle. Kissing and caressing are obvious preludes to sex, but they can be preceded by another aspect of foreplay, anticipation.
- The power of suggestion can be very strong. That's one of the merits of going for a romantic dinner for two. While the meal fulfils your hunger and thirst, gazing across the table at one another can whet your appetite for a different sort of dessert.
- When you do start canoodling, it can sometimes be more seductive to reveal your body slowly bit by bit rather than ripping off your clothes.
- Sexual anticipation can be built up gradually by gently stroking the less obvious erogenous zones, such as the thighs and feet.

The art of kissing

- The lips are one of the most sensitive parts of the body. As kissing is usually the first intimate act between new partners it's important to do it well, and good kissing is quite an art form.
- Don't keep your lips tightly puckered – loosen them up. The key is to vary kissing. Deep tongue penetration can be very erotic sometimes, while at others times try very soft nibbling.
- Due to its intimacy, kissing is often the first activity that stops when a relationship hits a bad patch.

Fantasy in foreplay

Almost everyone has sexual fantasies. For men, fantasising is typically used as an aid to arousal. Dreaming about someone other than your partner is common and shouldn't be regarded as a slight. Sometimes tiredness and other factors can inhibit your normal sexual response. On such occasions, running an imaginary blue movie through your mind does no harm if it helps you gain an erection. Foreplay is the most usual time for men to fantasise – during intercourse it can make the control of ejaculation difficult. It may not be a good idea to tell your partner about your fantasy – particularly if you've been thinking about her best friend.

Massage

The sex industry has given massage a bad name. But discounting its sleazy reputation, it's a great way to relax aching muscles and prepare the senses for sex.

Wake up your senses

- Massage can be a wonderfully relaxing activity in its own right or a highly stimulating type of foreplay. Each square inch of your skin contains about 15,000 nerve endings.
- A key benefit is that it relaxes those muscles that tighten up under the stresses and strains of modern life.
- Waking up your senses in this way is a great precursor to sex. It also serves to break down any unconscious barriers between you and your partner.

Massage techniques

Massage primarily involves stroking, kneading, and pummelling the muscles. The three massage types listed below involve broad, easy strokes to begin with, leading up to focus on the pressure points where tense muscles are at their tightest.

- Aromatherapy massage involves rubbing diluted essential oils into the skin. The aromatic molecules are absorbed into the body through its natural oil or sebum. It's particularly good for relieving tension.
- Enjoying a sensual massage (see p.124–125) with your partner is a good way to get to know one another's bodies, regardless of whether it leads on to having sex. Slow, rhythmic movements help to create a relaxed and intimate mood.
- Self-massage can enable you to avoid taking medication for a headache. Try rubbing the ridge between your neck and the back of your head for about 10 minutes, then rub your temples. Self-massage is also useful for easing aches and pains from sport or tension from work, such as neck and shoulder aches, which require you to reach around to rub and knead the afflicted areas. Tired thigh muscles can be relieved by gently kneading them with both thumbs. Tight hamstrings can be loosened by massaging with the backs of the fingers.

Practise massage skills

- It's best to get proper tuition in the art of massage, but there are some basic methods you can adopt. First, choose a warm, quiet location where you won't be disturbed.
- The subject should lie on a firm, flat surface, such as a firm bed. If the mattress is too soft, lay out a couple of blankets on the floor instead. The masseur should kneel on something comfortable if necessary. Drape towels over the parts of the body that are not going to be massaged.
- Use a light massage oil to reduce friction. Begin the massage with gentle, circular movements and try to keep to a constant rhythm. Small areas should be stroked with the thumbs and fingertips, whereas larger muscles can stand firmer pressure.

Massage benefits

- A massage need not take all night – but equally it should not be rushed. During the massage, concentrate on the hand movements and don't talk too much.
- A good massage should relax the muscles and the brain, inducing a pleasant weariness. Massages to specific parts of the body can have different effects. A foot massage can relax the whole body, for example, while a facial massage can ease headaches and leave your face feeling rejuvenated.

Essential oils for massage

Different essential oils for aromatherapy massage are widely regarded as having various therapeutic properties. A good choice for foreplay massage is an aphrodisiac oil that also has medicinal properties. Remember that neat essential oils must never be applied directly to the skin. They must be diluted first in neutral carrier oils. To add more diluted oil to the body, pour a little on to the back of the massaging hand first. The following are some popular massage oils: bergamot is uplifting and refreshing; lavender is refreshing, relaxing, and generally therapeutic; lemon grass is toning and refreshing; rosemary is invigorating; and ylang ylang is relaxing.

Sensual massage

An all-over body massage is wonderfully relaxing and intimate. But for safety, don't eat or drink immediately before a massage, avoid inflamed skin, and stop if a pain worsens.

SHOULDERS AND NECK
Nearly everyone experiences tension in the shoulders and neck. Lie your partner on her back and slide your fingers behind the neck and shoulders to gently massage this area.

BACK
Slowly stroke the back for relaxation, then move on to more stronger kneading and circling in particularly tense areas, such as underneath the shoulder blades.

ABDOMEN
Great sensitivity is required in when massaging this area. Smooth, gentle strokes in a clockwise direction can help relieve digestive problems.

HANDS AND ARMS
Arm muscles are usually quite strong so your movements can be firmer when massaging them.

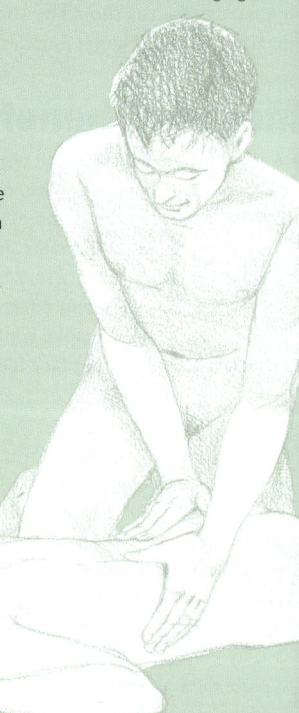

LEGS
Firm, repetitive massage of the legs stimulates the circulation, dispels fatigue, and helps relieve stiffness after exercise.

FEET
To avoid tickling your partner use firm movements and just enough oil to allow your fingers to move freely.

Different strokes

There are three basic types of massage stroke: stroking (also called "effleurage"), pressing ("petrissage"), and percussion. If you master these basic strokes, you can use them all over your partner's body to give her a relaxing and sensual full-body massage – then hope she returns the favour.

Stroking
This is the most basic stroke. It involves long, sweeping strokes with the palms of the hands. It's ideal for large body areas, like the back. Pressure can be either light or firm, or a mixture of the two.

Pressing
This stroke uses kneading movements. The flesh is gently squeezed, twisted, and rolled between the hands, fingers, and thumbs. It's used on muscles and joints that are tense, such as in the shoulders.

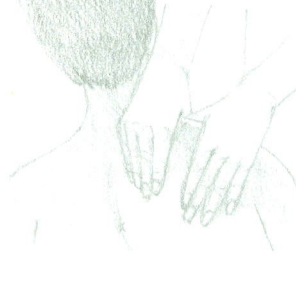
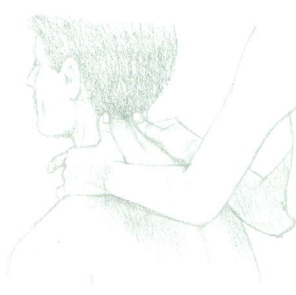

Percussion
This involves loosely cupping the hands and chopping the skin. It's a hacking motion that can be fast or slow and hard or soft. It's used on the more padded areas of the body.

Oral sex

Oral sex is extremely intimate and she likes it as much as you. So if you want her to keep doing that thing with her tongue, you'd better lick your own licking skills into shape.

Overcoming apprehension

- Despite the immense pleasure that both men and women get from oral sex, there can be considerable apprehension about the act on both sides.
- Some women fear that their genitals will smell or taste bad and are reluctant to allow their partner to go down on them. Such fears can be allayed by keeping the body clean and washing away stale odours.
- Some men are more than happy to receive oral sex but less keen to give it. This is not a helpful attitude, and may inhibit a woman's ability to relax and enjoy the experience if she feels her partner is giving her cunnilingus under duress.

Skill and responsiveness

- Learning how to be good at cunnilingus can take a little practise. Don't make the mistake of going straight for the genitals. Instead, work your way down her body, gently kissing and licking the stomach and thighs.
- Try to sense how relaxed your partner is. If she seems slightly tense, take your time and wait until her body unwinds. Licking gently, gradually move towards the outer labia (lips) and then the inner labia and the vagina.
- Finally move to the erotic epicentre of her body, the clitoris. Lick it very softly at first as it is packed with nerve endings and can be very sensitive.
- Many woman find it easier to achieve orgasm through oral sex than intercourse because it directly stimulates the clitoris. By listening to your partner's responses and by gradually increasing the pace of licking, you should be able to bring her to orgasm.
- Orgasm need not be the goal of cunnilingus; it's a highly effective foreplay technique, which prepares the body for sex.

Top ten tips for cunnilingus

1. **Take time** Your partner will enjoy oral sex most if she's completely relaxed. This is not an activity to be done in a hurry.

2. **Vary your technique** There are ways to vary how you give oral sex so try different techniques and see how your partner responds. If you don't know how comfortable your partner feels about cunnilingus, ask her.

3. **Edge your way** Start by kissing and licking the outer lips then the inner lips of her genitals.

4. **Take care with the cherry** At first, lick the clitoris gently. It's packed with nerve endings and is extremely sensitive.

5. **Vaginal fullness** Some women like to the have the tongue inserted into the vagina, stimulating intercourse. Alternatively, insert your finger or, better still, a dildo into the vagina while continuing to lick the clitoris.

6. **Building up** Slowly build up a rhythm by lapping at the vulva (external genitals) as if it were an ice cream. Use the tip of the tongue to make light flicks and the whole of the tongue to make broader licks. After a while, concentrate on licking alternate sides of the clitoris, but don't break your rhythm.

7. **Be patient** No matter how good you are, she's not going to climax straight away – listen to her breathing for signs.

8. **Persevere** Your tongue may ache, but you can reduce this by not stretching it out too far or licking too vigorously.

9. **Take care** Some sexually-transmitted diseases can be passed on by oral sex. Giving oral sex to a woman suffering from gonorrhea can lead to painful inflammation of the throat. Avoid giving cunnilingus if you have a cold sore.

10. **Mutual oral sex** The "69" position, in which one partner kneels above the other facing the other way, is an exciting variation, but some couples can find it difficult to fully enjoy the pleasures of receiving oral sex while continuing to give it.

The female genitals

- The collective term for the external female genitals is the vulva. The fleshy bit at the front of the genital area covered with hair is known as the pubic mound. The outer vaginal lips – the labia majora – are full and fleshy during a woman's reproductive years. These and the inner lips (labia minora) surround the highly erogenous clitoris.
- For many women, stimulation of the clitoris is an essential pre-requisite for an orgasm, either during sex or masturbation.

What you need to know

The vulva consists of the outer and inner labia, the clitoris, and the entrances to the vagina and urethra (through which she urinates). The outer labia majora are hairy on the outside and contain sweat glands on the inside. Within them are the labia minora, which encase the clitoris and the vaginal and urethral entrances. They contain secretory glands that prepare the genitals for intercourse. The visible part of the clitoris consists of a pinkish bud, but internally there is a mass of erectile tissue. The vagina has more sensory nerve endings towards the entrance, so large penises don't make that much of an extra impression.

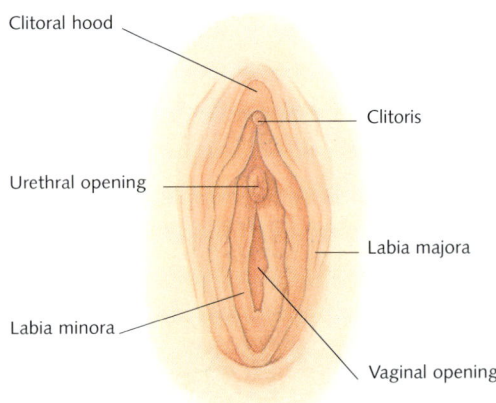

Fellatio

- For the average man, being given oral sex is one of life's greatest pleasures. The only mystery is why fellatio wasn't one of the words you were taught in Latin lessons at school.
- The word is Latin and means "sucking", but this isn't really a very accurate term. Oral sex is more likely to involve a woman licking a man's penis and testicles as well. The vast majority of men enjoy being given fellatio.
- It can also involve her taking the penis into her mouth and thrusting it in and out in a simulation of intercourse. It is, of course, a very intimate act. The sensation of your partner's soft moist mouth encasing your penis can be immensely exciting.

Give gentle directions

- It may seem obvious to you what's required. And indeed many women say they enjoy giving fellatio because it's an arousing activity for them as well as for you. But sometimes a little guidance may help the less experienced woman.
- Unlike the clitoris, the penis can stand a good deal of pressure. If your partner's oral administrations are a little too delicate, tell her. But be aware that some women can feel uncomfortable about tasting the part of your body that is used to urinate. Others may feel discomfort if the penis is thrust too deeply into the mouth.
- Then there's the matter of whether your partner wants to spit or swallow. There's no medical reason not to ejaculate into your partner's mouth if she's willing, unless you have an infection. But a lot of woman are not too keen on the taste of semen and prefer to pull away before ejaculation. There's no truth in the old myth that a woman can become pregnant by swallowing her partner's semen.

The advantages

- Fellatio is a great type of foreplay or a good alternative to penetrative sex. It can also be particularly useful for men with erection difficulties as it is a great stimulus for encouraging blood to flow into the penis.
- Many men simply enjoy being able to relax without feeling any pressure to perform.

Sexual phases

Doing what comes naturally is all well and good, but understanding what's happening during intercourse will give you more control – and more enjoyment for you and your partner.

The four stages of response

- **Excitement** The first sign of arousal is usually an erection with associated increases in heart rate, blood pressure, and muscle tension. Your partner's clitoris and labia swell and her vagina lubricates.
- **Plateau** The length of the plateau depends on the levels of sexual arousal. You both may develop a "sex flush". A small amount of pre-ejaculate fluid is emitted from your burgeoning penis. The clitoris enlarges but can become concealed by the swollen vaginal lips. The vaginal opening narrows, tightening its grip on the penis.
- **Orgasm** The prostate gland releases fluids that mix with sperm. Ejaculation occurs as rapid muscle contractions force semen out of the penis. Her orgasm consists of rapid involuntary spasms in the pelvic region.
- **Resolution** The heart rate of both you and your partner decreases and breathing returns to normal.

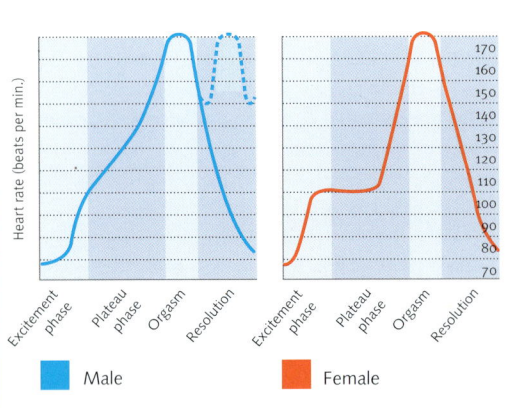

Brain power

- Although your penis may seem to have a mind of its own, your brain remains in charge during sex.
- It controls all the body's sexual responses, from the flush you may have on your cheeks to that tightening feeling in your scrotum as your testicles are pulled in closer to your body.
- The brain also operates on an emotional level during sex. It can boost your sexual response if you're flagging by thinking passionate thoughts about your partner or even running X-rated fantasies through your mind.
- Sometimes our thoughts can trouble us during sex. The brain may dredge up outdated negative messages that stem from our upbringing, such as the "sex is dirty" classic.
- Other anxieties may include fears about Aids, about making your partner pregnant, or about not being a good lover. Or there may be a voice at the back of your mind that says you shouldn't have got into bed with your partner in the first place. Such nagging worries can be inhibiting enough to wilt your erection.

Top tips for making it last

1. **Masturbate first** Younger men, in particular, can find it difficult to delay ejaculation. One possible solution – albeit rather crude – is to masturbate before sex. Many men find that this makes it easier to last longer.

2. **Choose your position** Some sexual positions are less stimulating for the man, notably when the woman is on top.

3. **Think positive** Sex therapists suggest that the way to prolong sex is to relax and enjoy it, rather than to allow an anxiety about premature ejaculation to trigger it off.

4. **Stop it** You can defer orgasm by temporarily stopping sex: withdraw from the vagina, change positions, or stimulate your partner manually for a while.

5. **Muscle control** Control the pubococcygeal muscles at the base of the scrotum. You use these to cut off the flow of urine and they can be trained to "squeeze off" orgasms.

Male orgasms

You know you like having an orgasm. The desire to climax is one of man's most powerful drives. But do you know what happens and how to make it feel even better?

The two stages

- The first stage involves sperm being drawn up from the testicles and mixed with seminal fluid from the prostate gland. You have a strong feeling that you're about to have an orgasm.
- The second stage is ejaculation, which usually occurs with orgasm. Muscles in the penis convulse rhythmically, pumping semen out of the end of your penis. There are usually three to five contractions, occurring at regular intervals of 0.8 seconds.

What happens when you orgasm

Sperm is carried from the testicles through the vas deferens to an area at the base of the urethra where it mixes with fluid from the prostate gland to become semen. Muscles close off the bladder from the urethra to ensure urine does not flow into the semen. Penis muscles contract rhythmically propelling the semen along the urethra.

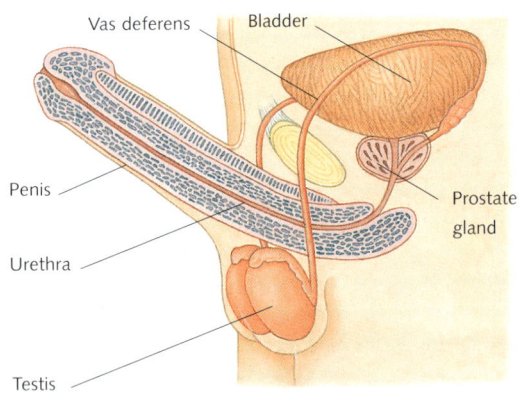

A teaspoon of sperm

- The average volume of semen released during ejaculation is 5ml (1/8floz) – equivalent to about one teaspoonful.
- Each ejaculate contains between 100 million and 500 million sperm.
- Sperm makes up only a small proportion of what is actually ejaculated. The rest of the milky liquid comprises nutrients, including vitamins, minerals, and proteins, which help to nourish the sperm and protect it from acids that are produced by the vagina.
- A sperm has three parts – a head, a mid-portion, and a tail.
- The head contains the man's genetic information which, when combined with the mother's chromosomes, ensures the child inherits traits from both parents.
- The mid-portion is the motor. It converts nutrients in the semen into energy enabling the sperm to swim to the egg.
- The tail propels the sperm at an average speed of 3mm (1/8in) per minute.
- Recent research has suggested that there are different types of sperm, which work together as a team. So-called killer sperms attempt to destroy rival sperms from another man, while blocker sperms seek to patrol the entrance to the cervix to prevent rival sperms getting through. A third type, so-called family-planning sperms, are the only ones capable of fertilising an egg.

Keep your sperm healthy

- Don't smoke.
- Don't drink too much. In particular, avoid binge-drinking. Try not to consume more than three units of alcohol a day.
- Don't wear tight underwear or tight trousers.
- Don't have too many hot baths – it's better to keep your testicles cool.
- Eat lots of fruit and vegetables. These will supply your body with useful C and E vitamins and beta-carotene.
- Boost your zinc intake by at least 20mg a day with a multivitamin supplement or zinc pill.
- Try to be sure your drinking water is not contaminated by the toxin lead.
- Reduce the amount of stress in your life.

Female orgasms

Women don't generally climax as easily as men through intercourse. But with their ability to have multiple orgasms, their potential enjoyment of sex may well surpass your own.

The female response

- As a woman starts to feel aroused, the vagina and clitoris become engorged with blood. The breasts also become larger and the nipples become erect.
- As the woman enters the plateau phase (see p.130), the vaginal muscles tighten to increase their grip on the penis and the clitoris may become concealed from view by the swollen labia (sometimes causing confusion for the male). From this point the woman may move on to the orgasm phase or not achieve orgasm and move straight to the resolution stage.
- An orgasm begins with rhythmic contractions in the vagina and then in the uterus. These movements are thought to help draw sperm towards the uterus and the fallopian tubes.
- Depending on the intensity of the orgasm, women usually experience between five and 15 orgasmic contractions, lasting up to about 15 seconds at the most.
- It's common for the back to arch and for the face to contort. Some women make noises and others make no sound at all.

Physiological similarities

A woman's orgasmic response mirrors that of a man in many ways. The orgasmic contractions occur at the same 0.8 second intervals and, as with a man's orgasm, the intensity of a woman's contractions diminishes rapidly after the first few, although the strongest female orgasms can be more long-lasting. The more intense climaxes also produce a greater total body reaction. A woman's heart rate can rise to 180 beats a minute. The muscles throughout her body, notably in the back and feet, may clench involuntarily, just as they do in a man.

Don't be all at "c"

- Many women find it difficult to achieve orgasm on a regular basis through penile penetration alone. This is because many sexual positions do not provide sufficient direct stimulation of the clitoris.
- With its mass of nerve endings, the clitoris is the erogenous centre of a woman's body. During masturbation, a woman stimulates the clitoral area for as long as she likes and in any way she prefers until she reaches orgasm.
- Rubbing and licking of the clitoris is, therefore, an important part of foreplay. Manual stimulation by either partner can continue during intercourse, so increasing the woman's likelihood of having an orgasm.
- Alternatively, the clitoris can be stimulated to a climax before or after intercourse.
- Locating this vitally female body part is a problem for many men (see p.128). Far from being a holy grail, this little pink bud is in fact neatly situated within the outer labia above the entry to the vagina. But don't feel ashamed if you can't find it – just ask for a little guidance.

The G-spot

- Named after a German gynaecologist called Grafenburg, the G-spot is said to be an extremely erogenous zone about 5cm (2in) up on the front wall of the vagina.
- The existence of the G-spot is still not a medically recognised fact, and it may be that it's only present in some women. But it has been claimed that pressure on this spot prompts an urge to urinate, followed by sexual arousal. This is said to lead in some cases to engorgement of the G-spot and then orgasm.
- These vaginal climaxes are thought to centre on the uterus, whereas clitoral orgasms are believed to be based on the contraction of the pubococcygeal (PC) muscles, which form part of the floor of the pelvic cavity.
- One of the best sexual positions for the stimulating the G-spot is said to be that of kneeling rear-entry (see p.178–179), as the angle of love-making brings the penis into direct contact with this allegedly super-sensitive part of the vaginal wall.

Moving the earth

As George Orwell didn't quite say: all orgasms are equal, but some are more equal than others. Follow these tips and your climax can be more of a rocket than a sparkler.

Top tips for intensifying orgasm

1 **Make sex last longer** The longer you hold off having an orgasm, the more powerful it's likely to be.

2 **Control your orgasmic response** Practise getting close to orgasm during sex and then backing off before you reach the point of so-called ejaculatory inevitability. This may mean you stop thrusting for a while until your excitement decreases. The disadvantage of stopping for a while is that it can interrupt your partner's growing level of arousal.

3 **Try new positions** Some positions offer much greater stimulation of the penis than others.

4 **Strengthen your PCs** Strong pubococcygeal muscles can mean more powerful orgasms (see p.139).

5 **Vent your feelings** Let your voice mirror what you're feeling by moaning, groaning, or yelling. Expressing yourself in this way will help you focus on your feelings.

6 **Go without** By going for several days without ejaculating, you'll build up a store of sperm and develop a strong sex drive. But such desire can make men prone to climaxing quicker than usual. The skill is, therefore, to control desire for as long as possible to ensure a strong orgasm.

7 **Get connected** Make sure the person in bed with you is someone you want to be having sex with! Sleazy one-night stands can be exciting – or they can be surprisingly boring. The strongest orgasms usually occur with someone you feel a close emotional connection with.

The ultimate orgasm

There often seems to be so much pressure to be good in bed that many people regard sex as a test rather than a pleasure. Men worry that they are climaxing too soon and not satisfying their partners, while women tend to worry that they are slow to climax. Both partners should learn to relax more and focus on their bodily sensations.

- Don't restrict movements, breathing, or the noise you make.
- Both partners should absolve one another of the oppressive requirement to deliver an orgasm.
- Sometimes, ejaculation may not always be the most pleasurable moment. Strong muscle contractions in the pelvis before and after the climax can be even more satisfying.
- Pursuing the ultimate orgasm can be regarded as somewhat selfish, as doing what feels best for you may compromise what's best for your partner. One solution may be for both of you to be more assertive in bed and to ask for what you want.

The importance of afterplay

- Don't think that sex ends with your orgasm. Being a good lover means developing something many men are not very good at – afterplay.
- Not only are women generally slower to become aroused and to reach orgasm, they are also slower to cool down after sex.
- Considering how much emotional involvement most women put into sex it figures that they also find it harder than men to disengage from the act.
- So, however sated and weary you may feel after ejaculation, show your love and appreciation for your partner by kissing, hugging, and generally remaining very close to her.
- The period straight after sex is also a good time to offer words of support to your partner. It's not a good time to make any criticisms. If there's something critical you want to point out leave it until another, less intimate, time when your partner won't take it as an instant rebuke of her sexual performance.

Multiple orgasms

Women may still be fighting for equal rights, but on the orgasm front they can do better than you. Yet some experts claim men can also train themselves to have multiple orgasms.

How to prolong pleasure

- All women have the capability to experience multiple orgasms, although achieving them is another matter.
- There's no secret recipe, but making sex last longer and being totally relaxed are keys. Your partner will feel more able to completely relax if she knows you can make love to her for at least 20 minutes without climaxing.
- Research shows that women in their thirties and forties are more likely to experience multiple orgasms, largely because they have become more relaxed and at ease with their bodies.

Multiple orgasms facts

- Only half of women surveyed claim to have experienced a multiple orgasm.
- 39 percent of 40-year-old women regularly have a single orgasm during sex compared with 30 percent of 20-year-olds.
- What is a multiple orgasm? One view claims it's a prolonged single orgasm, another claims it's a succession of orgasms.

Ejaculation and orgasm: the difference

A distinction can be made between male ejaculation and orgasm. Ejaculation is the emission of semen, with sensations confined to the genital area – essentially a mechanical function. In some men, particularly young men, it's possible to climax with minimal stimulation. Orgasm, on the other hand, can be described as a total-body experience. It generally requires a slow and steady build-up and, often, a strong emotional involvement. There's no debate about which is the most satisfying.

How to prolong pleasure

- Some experts claim that men can also learn to experience multiple orgasms. They say that with practise a man can enjoy the sensation of climaxing without actually ejaculating. In this way it's said you can have more than one orgasm.
- First, you need to gain control over your pubococcygeal (PC) muscles with a programme of exercises (see below). Second, you need to identify stages of sexual arousal so you can put the PC muscles to work at the right time (see p.130–131).

Waterworks training

- The pubococcygeal (PC) muscles are the ones you use to cut off the flow of urine when you pee.
- Exercises to improve these muscles are named after a gynaecologist called Arnold Kegel. The value of the Kegel exercises is that as well as enabling you to "squeeze off" an ejaculation – thereby paving the way for multiple orgasms – you can also gain firmer erections and stronger orgasms.
- Do the following exercises every day for about 6 weeks to get your PCs in top condition:

1. Contract and release your PC muscles quickly 10 times.

2. Contract and hold your PCs for 15 seconds.

3. Gradually increase this programme so that you are doing 10 sets of both steps one and two every day.

4. Do these exercises in different positions, such as on your stomach or your back.

Will it work?

- Unfortunately, there's no medical confirmation that men can have multiple orgasms. Indeed, some sex therapists believe the pursuit of them is misguided and can put men under extra pressure. But if having stronger PC muscles can help you to prolong your lovemaking, that can be a worthy goal in itself.
- Whatever you do try to achieve, make sure you keep your partner informed.

Alternatives to intercourse

Vaginal sex isn't the only way. Sometimes there are occasions when normal intercourse isn't desirable. The good news is there are lots of other ways to have satisfying sex.

How about outercourse?

- Sexual contact of any type can be very enjoyable and there are a number of alternatives to vaginal penetration.
- The term most commonly used by sex therapists to describe these alternatives is the rather cheesy-sounding "outercourse".
- In an era of Aids and other sexually-transmitted diseases, one of the many advantages of outercourse is obvious (remember though that oral sex can cause disease to spread).
- Sex therapists and experts point to several other reasons why outercourse can sometimes be preferable to penetrative sexual intercourse:

No babies There's no chance of pregnancy if sperm is kept out of the vagina. This means no contraception, and hence no risk of side effects from pills or chemicals.

No erection required Outercourse is good for men who may be having problems getting and maintaining an erection. It has been suggested that you don't have to have an erection to enjoy sex. Stimulation of the flaccid penis can also feel good. This can relieve a lot of the pressure on men who feel anxious about their performance.

During menstruation Although there's no physical reason not to continue having sex during a woman's period, some couples are uncomfortable with penetrative sex at this time.

During pregnancy Women often experience changes in their sex drive during pregnancy – sometimes for more sex, sometimes for less. If penetration becomes uncomfortable, outercourse is a good alternative. Non-penetrative sex is also a good way to begin to re-establish intimacy after the birth of a child, when intercourse may still be painful.

Exploring the alternatives

BODY RUBBING
Resourceful couples can find ways of relieving a man's sexual desire without the pregnancy risk of intercourse. One of the most popular ways is to rub your penis against those parts of your partner's body that provide enough friction to bring you to orgasm.

The most popular place is probably between the breasts. For many men this is enough of an attraction irrespective of concerns about contraception. Another good place to rub your penis is between your partner's thighs, either from the front or behind. Similar stimulation can also be gained under your partner's armpits.

ANAL INTERCOURSE
In the days before reliable contraception was available, anal sex was regarded as a good alternative to vaginal intercourse because it avoided the risk of pregnancy. These days it's practised by some heterosexual couples, mainly because of the unusual sensations it can provide. Deep penetration can be very painful for a woman; one problem being that the anus does not produce its own lubrication. Friction can make the tissues of the rectum tear easily, causing bleeding. This gives sexually transmitted diseases, such as HIV and hepatitis, a direct route into the bloodstream.

For these reasons it's essential to wear an extra-strong condom and to use a water-based lubricant (oil-based lubricants destroy condom rubber). To avoid the risk of infection, be absolutely certain to wash your hands and penis after contact with your partner's anus before touching her vagina.

Some couples prefer to avoid anal penetration and stimulate the anal hot spots by stroking around the anus and perineum instead.

MUTUAL MASTURBATION
You can stimulate one another simultaneously or take it in turns. A variation is to watch one another as you masturbate yourselves.

Games and fantasies

Usual bedroom routine getting boring? Try spicing it up with games – and we're not talking chess. With any luck, you'll both be more than happy when she's got the whip in hand.

Why play games?

- Even the best of relationships can sometimes go stale and require a bit of spice in the sex department. These could range from strip poker or talking dirty to more elaborate scenarios, such as role-playing and gentle bondage.
- The key with such activities is for both partners to be completely happy with what's going on at all times. Since the objective is to bring you closer together, it's no use demanding that your partner performs acts that she finds distasteful.
- Be careful when broaching the subject. The best time to say you might like to whip her is not when she's feeling vulnerable, but at a neutral time, such as while on a walk. And make it clear that what you're suggesting is just that – a suggestion.

Flights of fantasy

Almost everyone has sexual fantasies. It may be true that men think about sex more often, but there's now greater recognition that women also enjoy reading and watching sexually explicit material. Both sexes often fantasise during love-making to enhance their sexual pleasure without telling their partners. Many men have a catalogue of explicit thoughts stored away, often involving having sex with another woman, watching a lesbian love scene, or taking part in an orgy. Some people feel guilty about such thoughts, believing they are being disloyal to their partner. But as long as a fantasy remains distinct from enacting it out in real life, there'll be no harm done. One way to enhance a relationship is to share fantasies. But tread carefully. You might like to start by reading erotic stories instead.

Feed your imagination

Fantasy games add variety to a relationship that may have become routine. Many relationship or sex therapists say that such games can keep couples together by creating harmony and reducing lustful desires to have sex with other people. In terms of fantasies and role-playing, men are more likely to imagine themselves as the dominant partner, while women tend to envisage scenarios in which they are subservient in some way. But this isn't always the case. Some men have a desire to be dominated and told what to do, while some women also fantasise about having a male sex slave. Whatever you and your partner want to do to pep up your sex can almost certainly be enacted. The only proviso is that you both have an implicit understanding of the acceptable limits of behaviour. Try some of these:

MISTRESS AND SERVANT
The lady of the house has strong demands and you must do her bidding.

SEDUCER AND STRANGER
Arrange to arrive at a bar separately and use all your charm to seduce that beautiful woman in the corner. But make sure it is your partner.

PLAYING INNOCENT
Many men like their partner to enact the role of the innocent virgin. This can make you feel the sexual master you've always wanted to be, while both of you can revive memories of the first time you had sex together all those years ago.

MASKS AND COSTUMES
Masks can add a certain kinkiness to proceedings. But be sure that your partner is happy with you wearing a Dracula or Batman outfit – she may not like it if it serves to act as a barrier between you, and you may run the risk of making her laugh.

A bit of bondage

- Many couples enjoy a little light bondage. This involves one person being restrained in some way, usually by having the hands or legs tied together or tied to bed posts or other furniture. Useful restraining items include bathrobe cords, bed sheets, or anything else that doesn't hurt.
- We're not talking about serious bondage here. It's a good idea for you and your partner to discuss the boundaries of what you both think is acceptable before trying anything new in this particular area of sex play.
- But equally, if you have complete trust in each other, it can be enjoyable to allow your partner to tie you up and lead you into an area of uncharted dominance.
- The attraction of bondage is that one partner surrenders unconditionally while the other gains total control of the situation. This creates an unusual psychological power scenario quite in contrast to the mutuality of regular love-making. Sex psychologists say that people who have a repressed attitude to sex, perhaps because of their upbringing, enjoy being "forced" into submission because it frees them from any sense of guilt they may feel about having sex.

Bondage essentials

- **Restraining** Good items for tying the hands include silk scarves, pillow cases, and handkerchiefs – anything that won't dig into the skin. Whatever you use, don't tie it so tightly that it becomes uncomfortable.
- **Blindfolds** To enhance the role of the submissive, wrap a scarf or hand towel around the head to act as a blindfold for increasing anticipation.
- **Whip** A riding crop is the ideal whip but you could improvise with anything else from around the house, such as some cord or a long, supple twig from the garden.
- **PVC** Black leather or PVC clothing is probably the most erotic of the female corrective uniforms. Thigh-length boots and high heels complete the get-up. But make sure your partner will be happy to wear them before you splash out on such purchases.

A popular pastime

- Sado-masochism (S&M) is an increasingly popular form of sexual activity. Sadism is the practice of enjoying giving some form of intense stimulation to your partner, perhaps involving a degree of pain in some cases, while masochism is about enjoying being on the receiving end of such stimulation.
- While yet to enter the mainstream of sexual activity, S&M has come to be regarded as more acceptable and less marginalised than it used to be. The practice focuses on "discipline" as a form of erotic punishment, usually involving caning or spanking.
- Sensations of pain and pleasure are registered in the same area of the brain, which may explain the appeal of S&M.
- For most S&M participants, it's not about serious pain. The enjoyment comes from the body's (often the bottom's) ability to receive an enjoyable feeling of stimulation with mild pain.

Exploring the scene

- There's an extensive network of S&M clubs and activities around the UK. How much you and your partner want to get involved in this public scene is, of course, up to you. There are several societies catering to different aspects of bondage, dominance, and S&M, some of which publish magazines.
- There are also many clubs featuring S&M nights. These tend to have strict dress codes which require you to wear some form of fetish clothing. This is to deter non-participants who just want to watch.
- Some clubs are racier than others. It should be noted that the "rules" governing what goes on in S&M clubs may differ greatly from country to country.

Unwritten rules

- Whatever games you and your partner play, there are limits to what you should do. In some situations your partner may be putting her complete trust in you. Recognise that there are lines that should not be crossed.
- Practising S&M may demand a little more freedom of manner than you may be used to, but don't do anything that could cause either you or your partner shame or unacceptable pain.

Sexual aids

What are you anxious about? A sex toy can help her achieve orgasm and take the pressure off you to perform. Get up to speed with a vibrator and you'll have her purring with delight.

A potted history

Sex aids have been used for thousands of years:
- Greek dildos. It is not known who created the dildo, but ladies in ancient Greece certainly used them. The name dildo probably comes from the Italian word *diletto* in the Renaissance era, which means to delight. Early models were fairly crude. Made of wood or leather, they needed plenty of lubrication with olive oil to be comfortable for use. Rubber dildos did not appear until the 19th century.
- Chinese rings. The ancient Chinese would tie silk around the base of the penis to help maintain an erection. They also devised a feathered ring which, when inserted over the penis, helped to tickle the woman to orgasm.
- Vibrators. The first vibrators, made in the second half of the 19th century, were thinly disguised as medical devices. They were used to treat hysteria, the term used in the Victorian era to describe women suffering from sexual fantasy and heavy vaginal lubrication. Physicians used vibrators to bring the "patient" to orgasm.

Bedroom essentials

For nights of varied passion, a well-equipped bedroom should have a good supply of the following items:
Condoms These can be used as sex toys as well as for contraception.
Lubrication Make sure you only use water-based products. Oil-based lubricants can erode condoms and cause inflammation of the penis and vagina.
Massage oil Try blends of nut and vegetable oils.
Silk scarves Ideal for tying one another up.

The classics

Vibrators Vibrators are probably the most popular sex toys and the most suitable for use by couples. When pressed against a woman's clitoris, labia, and nipples the vibrations given off enable most women to achieve an orgasm.
Mostly made of plastic or metal, vibrators come in various shapes and sizes and operate by battery or are plugged into the mains.
The speed of vibration is important. Choose a vibrator which offers various speeds. As well as great fun during foreplay, vibrators can also be used during lovemaking to stimulate your partner's clitoris. But the fun isn't just for your partner. Men, too, enjoy the feeling of vibration, particularly around the penis and anus.

Dildos Dildos tend to be more realistically shaped like penises than vibrators, but without the vibrating action. They are used as artificial penises during masturbation or gay sex.
Dildos are available in a wide range of shapes and sizes, and some have a base which can be filled with water and squeezed to simulate ejaculation.

Cock rings Cock rings fit around the base of the penis to help maintain erection by trapping blood inside the penis. They should not be worn for prolonged periods.

Love balls These are small metal or plastic balls that are inserted into the vagina for extended periods. As the woman moves around the balls move around inside her, generating erotic sensations. Battery-operated vibrating eggs can be also used and switched on to increase the sensation. Some models have a remote control switch so you can take your partner by surprise and perhaps make a trip to the supermarket more interesting.

Clitorial stimulators These are small rings that fit around the base of the penis and have a small protrusion that rubs against the clitoris during sex.

Dressing for sex

Your choice of underwear is rich in erotic significance. Dating your dream woman may come to nothing if stripping off your designer clothes reveals tent-sized Y-fronts.

The fundamentals

- Whether you're fashion-fixated or a dowdy dresser, there are principles that all men should adhere to. Generally, you should clean your clothes regularly. Dirty clothes suggest that you are dirty and that you don't take good care of yourself.
- Clean underwear is essential. This means clean pants and socks every day – not fishing around in the laundry bin for the least dirty pair when you've run out. Whatever the state of your socks, they should always be removed before sex.

Choosing your underwear

- The main choice is between briefs and boxers. Briefs are popular as they do a better job of holding you in place, but some women prefer the looser look of boxer shorts. They also conceal unseemly bulges and allow more air to circulate around your genitals, keeping the testicles cooler.
- Old-style Y-fronts should only be worn if you deliberately wish to turn a woman off. A popular modern alternative is button-fronted cotton trunks.
- Check fabrics carefully – only buy 100 percent cotton or a cotton/lycra combination as man-made fabrics retain sweat, which encourages the growth of bacteria.

The passion killers

- Builder's bottom – sagging jeans are a major no-no.
- Flies undone – leave flying low to the fighter pilots.
- Smelly pits – good for making her faint, but certainly not with passion.
- Unclean pants – don't even think about it.
- Tight clothing – tight shirts and skin-tight trousers are not generally attractive sights.

Buying for your partner

- In contrast to men, women have a much wider choice of sexy underwear. But it should be borne in mind that while most women like to look desirable by wearing something sexy, most of these garments are devised by men to suit men's desires about what looks erotic on a woman. Peep-hole bras are just one example.
- Other classic sexy underwear includes stockings and suspenders, French knickers, and see-through panties. Many of these items are available in what are regarded as erotic fabrics and materials, such as silk, leather, and rubber – these are generally preferable to synthetic materials which can scratch or look cheap.

Do some research

- You may think your partner would look fantastic in black rubber, but are you sure she would be comfortable wearing it?
- Buying erotic underwear can be a bit of a minefield. Some women feel that they must be undesirable if their partner takes it upon himself to buy them something sexy to wear. And many men fail to appreciate that buying sexy underwear is as much a present to themselves as to their partners. Women can feel a little cheated by such "gifts".
- If you're confident your partner will be a willing recipient, make sure you know her size and what colours she would like to wear before you go shopping. Far too many men wander into shops, struggle to remember their partner's sizes, and end up making vague comparisons with shop assistants.

Brace yourself

- If all this sounds too daunting, you could buy goods by mail order or over the internet.
- Better still, why not go shopping with your partner? That way you can choose her clothes you both like and she'll be able to try them on. In fact, there's less chance you'll feel like a dirty old man when wandering around the racks of lacy bras and crotchless panties in her company rather than by yourself.
- The only danger is that your partner may spot some awful pair of thongs that she thinks might look good on you.

Potency

As a hormonally-charged teenager, your main problem was controlling that miscreant below your belt. But as you get older, the stresses of life can inhibit your ability to rise to the occasion. Here's how to cope...

Use it or lose it

- There is evidence to suggest that having sex regularly ensures that you'll want to continue having sex.
- Making love regularly stimulates the production of testosterone, which in turn fuels the male sex drive.
- Also, keep yourself in good shape. The fitter you are, the more you'll be able to cope with work pressures and stress, thereby minimising their impact on your sex drive.
- For a healthy sexual appetite, watch what you eat and make sure your only spare tyre is the one in the car.

Physical health and sex

- All sorts of psychological problems can affect a man's sex drive, but even the most relaxed and unstressed man can have a problem getting an erection if there's a physical impediment.
- Circulatory problems are often to blame. An erection can only be attained if blood is able to engorge the penis. So keep your circulatory system in good shape by working out and not smoking. Diabetics can suffer poor blood flow, but drinking too much alcohol and taking drugs are entirely avoidable.

Mental health and sex

- Stress can have a big impact on your sex life. If you've got worries about money or an illness, or if you fear your job may be under threat, your libido can fall significantly.
- Another form of stress is having too much work to do. If you go to bed with your brain churning over what you have to do the next day, you're unlikely to be in the right frame of mind to enjoy sex. Try to change your lifestyle to reduce stress. Failing that, at least practise some relaxation exercises.

Understanding testosterone

- Testosterone is a natural anabolic steroid hormone that's produced by the testicles. Levels of testosterone vary throughout a man's life, increasing markedly during puberty to prompt the physical changes that transform a boy into a man.
- For most men – about four out of every five – levels of testosterone stay within normal limits during their life, although the amount of the hormone in the blood declines gradually after the age of 50.
- Testosterone is responsible for maintaining the sex drive; the deepening of the voice; the growth of the penis, testes and scrotum; stimulating sperm production; maintaining the ability to ejaculate; and the upkeep of the body's muscle bulk.
- Testosterone affects male sexual behaviour. One study found that husbands with high levels of the hormone were more likely to have affairs, while those with lower levels were less likely to get divorced.

Sex drive drugs

There is no such thing as a normal sex drive. Men have a wide variety of libidos, and sexual desire rises and falls throughout life. But for men who have purely physiological problems, there are some types of prescriptive drugs that almost guarantee an erection:

- **Viagra** This was launched in the UK in 1998 and is available only on prescription. It's not a sex hormone or aphrodisiac. It works by increasing the blood flow to the penis. Viagra does not produce an erection of its own accord – the man must still be sexually stimulated. Some men have side effects, including headaches and stomach upsets, while a few have died of heart attacks. For this reason it is important that you discuss the suitability of taking the drug with your doctor.
- **Caverject** This is prescribed for impotence. The active ingredient, injected by the man into his penis, mimics a substance found in the body that helps keep blood vessels open and increases blood flow. Caverject is claimed to produce erections in 80 percent of all users.

Aphrodisiacs

Aphrodisiacs are named after the Greek goddess of love, Aphrodite, and describe substances that are said to heighten sexual desire.

Various foods, liquids, and drugs have been championed throughout history as having aphrodisiac properties. Claims have been made for a host of goods, including Spanish fly, fresh figs, ginger, and a wealth of unsavoury-sounding animal genitalia. Some foods have phallic overtones, such as bananas and powdered rhino horn, while others are symbolic of the female genitals, such as oysters and mussels.

Men have spent centuries searching for wonder substances that would make women want to have sex with them or that would boost their impotency:

- The Greeks favoured eggs, honey, snails, mussels, and crabs.
- The Chinese were keen on powdered products. One was a blend of powdered plant roots called the bald chicken drug, which was said to enable a man to keep 40 women satisfied.
- Another Chinese drug included liver from a dead white dog. When applied to the penis, the substance was said to make the male member grow.
- In India, the Kama Sutra advised men who wanted to win over a woman to mix white thorn apple, black pepper, and honey and smear it over the penis before intercourse.
- Pine nuts have been extolled for centuries. In Roman times, the poet Ovid wrote that the "nuts that the sharp-leaved pine brings forth" acted as an aphrodisiac.

Do they work?

While the scientific basis for many aphrodisiac claims is weak, one substance that does have a strong claim is yohimbine. It's the bark from an African tree of the same name, which prompts erections by dilating the blood vessels in the genitals. Other substances, such as hot spices, can have an aphrodisiac effect by raising the body temperature, mirroring what happens during sexual arousal. But the vast majority of so-called aphrodisiacs may only work if the consumer believes they will.

Aphrodisiacs under analysis

- **Animal genitalia** These have been touted as aphrodisiacs for centuries in the belief that consumption of a healthy animal organ might cure a problem in the corresponding human organ. Among the targets have been the genitals of deer, asses, and monkeys. In recent years there has been demand in China for the genitals of dead seals. In Taiwan, a bowl of tiger penis soup can fetch £200 regardless of the fact that tigers are endangered.
- **Asparagus** Its main appeal is its appearance. But one 19th-century writer pointed out that while it turned men on, it had the opposite effect on women.
- **Celery seeds** These are said to work as an aphrodisiac when crushed and used in spiced bread or on salads.
- **Ginseng** This is claimed to have stimulant properties that help keep you awake – which is, at least, one of the pre-requisites for sex.
- **Oysters** Oysters have been regarded as an aphrodisiac for several centuries. But if there's any basis for the claim, it may be that they feel very slippery and sensuous in the mouth. Other seafood, like lobsters, are also highly touted, as is chipi-chipi, a small Venezuelan clam.
- **Rhino horn** This is believed to help men gain an erection – with the result that all five rhino species are now on the endangered list. It's interesting to note that original claims were for the dried penis and not the horn. The horn is largely made of a protein called keratin, so you'd probably do just as well to eat a lump of cheese.
- **Snakes** These are consumed in eastern Asia to boost the male libido. Cobra appears to be the favourite type of snake, and the best effects are said to be had by drinking the blood fresh.
- **Spanish fly** This preparation is made from the crushed and dried bodies of a southern European beetle. Its traditional uses are as a counter-irritant for skin blisters and as a particularly effective sexual stimulant for older gentlemen wishing to regain their youthful potency.
- **Truffles** These were highly rated by the Romans for their alleged aphrodisiac properties, and they have since been championed by the French.

Dealing with impotency

The only shameful thing about being impotent is not seeking help. Erection problems affect most men at some time, and in most cases they can be overcome.

Impotency and age

- It's a big misconception that impotence is an inevitable part of ageing. It's true that the frequency and strength of a man's erection may decrease, but there's no reason why he shouldn't be able to perform sexually into his eighties and even beyond.
- The causes of erection problems are either psychological or physical, and it's usually easy to identify which of these it is.
- If a man wakes up with an erection or can masturbate to orgasm, the problem is more likely to be psychological.
- Common physical causes of impotence are fatigue and stress. Other physical inhibitors include disorders that limit blood flow to the penis, such as heart disease and diabetes, depression, hardening of the arteries, and medications that cause impotence as a side effect.

Is it in the mind?

- Psychological problems are estimated to account for just over half of all impotence cases. The problems can be very varied, ranging from boredom or guilt to anxiety or depression.
- Such problems can become a vicious circle – the more a man thinks he will not get an erection, the less likely it is to happen. A psychological problem can sometimes be prompted by a physical one. A one-off drunken failure to get an erection may become a source of anxiety on future sober occasions.
- The keys to overcoming impotence are learning to relax and having the support of your partner. A cruel jibe about your performance from your partner may have contributed to the problem initially, but the best course of action is to communicate about it.
- Don't get sucked into the habit of avoiding physical contact as it will consequently make your partner feel rejected. There are professional therapists who can help.

When to seek help

It's estimated that only about 10 percent of men with impotence seek professional help, which is a great shame. With the wide range of treatments now available, well over 90 percent of sufferers can regain the ability to get an erection and enjoy a sex life once more.

What help is available

- The drug Viagra has a high success rate (see p.151).
- The MUSE technique involves the insertion of a drug pellet into the end of the penis. It produces an erection in about two-thirds of cases by relaxing the muscles in the penis.
- In vacuum therapy, the penis is placed in a plastic cylinder from which the air is drawn out and blood engorges the penis.
- Injection therapy requires the self-injection of a substance, such as Caverject, into the shaft of the penis. This works by dilating the blood vessels in the penis.
- Penile implants involve the surgical insertion of semi-rigid rods. This solution should be regarded as a last resort.

Sensate focusing

- One way to deal with impotence is by practising sensate focus touching exercises with your partner. The key aspect is that sex is banned, so relieving pressure.
- Couples touch different parts of one another's bodies before moving on to breasts and genitals. The aim is to get to know the whole of one another's bodies rather than rushing to the major erogenous zones.
- This helps both partners to experience pleasure without feeling anxious that intercourse must inevitably follow.
- The last of the caressing exercises is mutual masturbation. The woman should touch and caress the penis but move her hand away if it starts to become erect. The idea is to get the man used to the feelings of arousal without the immediate pressure to have sex.
- After a period of time, these exercises can help many men overcome their impotence.

Contraceptive methods

It can be easy to forget that sex is actually about making babies. So if you don't want to hear the patter of tiny feet just yet, decide which of the many forms of contraception is best for you and your partner.

The female pill

- When taken correctly, the combined pill is said to be 99 percent effective in preventing pregnancy.
- The most common type of pill contains a combination of synthetic oestrogen and progesterone.
- The eggs in the ovaries are prevented from being released, thereby making it impossible for them to be fertilised. The combined pill also thickens the cervical mucus so that it becomes hostile to sperm. The development of the uterus lining is also disrupted so that any egg that does manage to be released and fertilised cannot be implanted.
- Women must take the pill every day in 21- or 28-day cycles.
- The combined pill can have some side effects, including headaches, nausea, mood swings, and an increase in blood pressure. There are also fears that it may be a cause of breast cancer.
- Another type of pill is called the mini-pill, which contains only synthetic progesterone. Its effectiveness depends on the woman taking it at exactly the same time every day, whereas there is slightly more leeway with the combined pill.

The morning-after pill

If you have unprotected intercourse – or if your condom bursts – your partner has two emergency contraception options. The first is the morning-after pill, which can actually be taken within 72 hours of unprotected sex. It can be obtained from your doctor or a family planning clinic. These pills work by stopping ovulation or by preventing a fertilised egg from implanting. They're not designed to be taken regularly. The second emergency option is for an intrauterine device (see next page) to be fitted within five days of intercourse.

The coil

- The coil is the common name for an intrauterine device (IUD). This is a plastic device, sometimes wrapped in copper wire, which is inserted in the uterus by a doctor.
- It works by making the uterus a hostile environment for sperm and by preventing fertilised eggs from implanting.
- A coil can remain in place for anything up to 10 years.
- Some types of coil also release small amounts of synthetic progesterone, which helps to stop sperm reaching the fallopian tubes.
- The downside of coils is that they can increase the chances of infections spreading to the pelvis. They also increase the chances of an ectopic pregnancy (when the fertilised egg grows in the fallopian tube and has to be surgically removed). Both pelvic infections and ectopic pregnancies can lead to permanent infertility.
- The coil is usually only recommended for women in stable relationships who are unlikely to pick up sexually transmitted infections and for women who have had children, as this makes it easier for the coil to be inserted.

The male pill

- Ever since the launch of the female pill in the 1960s there's been talk about developing a male equivalent. The female pill initiated a social revolution for women based on sexual freedom but it came with side effects.
- Many people think it would only be fair for men to shoulder some of the discomforts of a hormonal contraceptive. But it's estimated that less than 10 percent of all research and development spending is allocated for male contraceptives.
- One factor is that many women say they couldn't trust their partner to remember to take the pill every day.
- A major factor is physical: finding a way to stop the production of sperm. Research is focusing on injecting male hormones into the bloodstream, which could prompt the brain to generate fewer relevant hormones.
- Another challenge is to create a contraceptive that inhibits sperm production without affecting a man's sex drive. Research continues to explore these challenges, but at present the male pill remains on the drawing board.

Barrier methods

The condom and cap are called barrier contraceptives because they form physical barriers that stop sperm reaching the uterus.

A girl's best friend

- Worldwide, the condom is the most popular contraceptive. It presents no health risks or side effects and is regarded as the best barrier to sexually-transmitted diseases.
- When used correctly, it's a very reliable form of contraception, responsible for only two pregnancies a year when used by 100 couples as their only form of contraception.
- The only possible side effect is for men and women who develop an allergy to rubber or spermicide.
- Condoms are easy to carry, relatively cheap, and do not require a visit to a doctor or clinic. They're popular with women because men are shouldering some of the contraceptive burden.
- Some men complain that having to put a condom on can interrupt the flow of passion. With a little forward-planning, such as keeping the condoms beside the bed, this can be minimised. And while some men say condoms reduce sensitivity, this very feature can help others who are prone to premature ejaculation to last longer.
- They are no longer found only in chemist shops and barbers'.

Condom types

Condoms are made mostly from thin, pre-lubricated rubber in different thicknesses, colours, and textures. Be aware that some types of novelty condoms are not intended for contraception. Always look for brands that carry the British Standard Kitemark. To enhance female sensation, condoms with ridges and knobbles are available. A recent development is the plastic condom for those with rubber allergies, and it is claimed it causes less reduction in sensitivity during sex.

How to put on a condom

Put on a condom before the penis makes any contact with the vagina. Open the packet carefully to avoid tearing the condom.

1 Squeeze the teat of the condom to expel air with one hand and roll the condom down the penis with the other hand (don't unroll the condom before putting it on).
2 Roll the condom right down to the base of the penis to limit the possibility of it sliding off during intercourse or of semen escaping.

After ejaculation, hold the base of the condom in place and withdraw from the vagina while you still have the erection. This will ensure no semen is spilt.

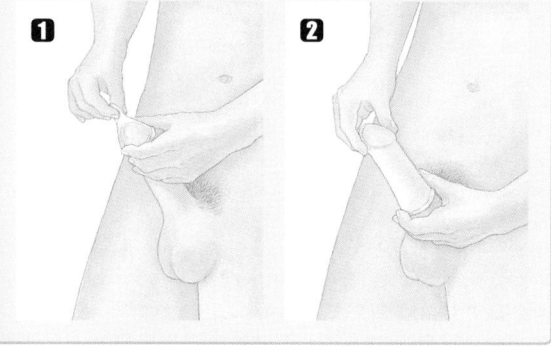

The dutch cap

- A cap (or diaphragm) is a dome of soft, thin rubber, which fits over the cervix up against the pubic bone. It works by blocking semen from passing through the cervix.
- A cervical cap is a smaller rubber device which fits over the opening of the uterus.
- Caps must first be fitted by a doctor, who will then show a woman how to fit it herself. Extra protection is gained by using a spermicidal jelly or cream. Both devices must stay in the vagina for at least six hours after sex to prevent any sperm from reaching the uterus. It's a chore for women to put them in, but they present very few health risks.

Natural methods

Natural methods of contraception, traditionally the preserve of Catholics, have also found favour among non-Catholics who want natural, drug- and barrier-free sex.

The rhythm method

- The rhythm method is a rather inexact science, which depends on not having sex when the woman is most likely to be fertile.
- It's based on working out the safe period during a woman's monthly cycle. This means identifying when ovulation occurs. After ovulation, the egg survives for no more than 24 hours. But because sperm can survive for up to 7 days in the fallopian tubes, you must not have sex in the week before ovulation.
- The problem is that most women who are not on the pill have variable menstrual cycles, which means it's difficult to predict when ovulation occurs. This makes working out the safe days during the first half of the cycle a somewhat hit and miss business.
- There are two main methods of pinpointing the date of ovulation. The temperature chart method involves the woman taking her temperature with a special thermometer every morning and plotting it on a fertility chart with great accuracy. It works on the basis that her temperature rises by about 0.5°C at ovulation. The safe phase is said to start when that higher temperature has been recorded for a third successive morning.
- The second method, sometimes called the Billings method, is to notice when the cervical mucus becomes thicker, which it does after ovulation. Both these methods require proper training by a family planning expert, preferably for you as well as your partner.
- The advantages of the rhythm method are that it's natural, it teaches you all about the menstrual cycle, costs nothing, and presents no health risks. The disadvantages are that it requires careful body monitoring and a large amount of will power.

Computerised contraception

- In 1996 the first computer-style contraception device was launched, which was touted as making temperature readings and mucus analysis a thing of the past.
- The device, known as a Persona, works out when ovulation is likely to occur by measuring the hormone levels in urine. The woman has to pee on a special stick, which is inserted into the devise. A series of green, amber, and red lights tells her when it is and isn't safe to have sex.
- The disadvantages are that it takes three months of programming to get to know a woman's monthly behaviour and its set-up is disrupted by use of either the regular hormonal pill or the emergency morning-after pill.
- More importantly, in spite of manufacturers' claims that the Persona is 96 percent reliable, there have been a significant number of unwanted pregnancies reported.
- This may be a good device to use if you and your partner are planning a pregnancy rather than trying to prevent one.

Mysteries of menstruation

- The average age at which a girl has her first period is 12, although the standard age range is 10–16.
- Women menstruate until they reach the menopause, normally in their late forties or early fifties. This means they are likely to have about 400 periods in total.
- About every 28 days, an ovary releases a mature egg. This passes down into the uterus where it may or may not be fertilised by sperm.
- If the egg is not fertilised, the lining of the uterus breaks down and is discharged through the vagina. This menstrual period marks the start of the menstrual cycle.
- The female cycle has nothing to do with the moon. Women's cycles can be as short as 16 days or as long as 40 days. The only concerning factor is that the periods are reasonably regular and do not involve excessive blood loss.
- Some women are more affected than others by the symptoms of premenstrual tension (PMT). These occur in the days leading up to menstruation and can include emotional angst, depression, headaches, tearful outbursts, and fatigue.
- There is no medical reason to avoid having sex during a period.

Surgical methods

Surgical sterilisation is a means of permanently preventing pregnancy. The male operation is relatively simple, but choosing to have a vasectomy is still a very big decision.

Vasectomy

- The vas deferens (the two tubes that carry the sperm from the testicles to the urethra) are surgically cut or tied.
- Vasectomy does not affect ejaculation, it just means there's no sperm in the semen. There is a reversal operation, but it's not always successful and a vasectomy should be regarded as a permanent operation.
- Some men take out a sort of insurance by depositing sperm in a private sperm bank.

The procedure

- A vasectomy can be performed under a local or general anaesthetic. It usually takes about 15 minutes, is relatively painless (most men report a pulling sensation in the abdomen), and most men return to non-strenuous work within a day.
- Some newer techniques involve the injection of a substance that forms a plug to block the vas deferens tubes.

Pros and cons

- Vasectomy is regarded as a minor operation.
- It rarely requires an overnight stay in hospital.
- The only discomfort may be slight tugging or bruising.
- You can have sex again as soon as any discomfort wears off – often within a day or two. But the first few ejaculations can feel slightly painful.
- There should be no effect on orgasm or ejaculation.
- Some men may experience impotence in the misguided belief that the operation has left them castrated.
- Vasectomy can take up to 3 months to be effective.

Female sterilisation

- Like a vasectomy, female sterilisation is difficult to reverse and should be regarded as permanent.
- It's popular with older women who feel they've had enough children, or who are worried about passing on an hereditary disease.
- After sterilisation, a woman continues to ovulate but the egg, instead of reaching the uterus, can get no further than the fallopian tubes. There it comes to a stop and dies.
- A hysterectomy is the most extreme form of female sterilisation involving the removal of the uterus. It's a major operation that makes it impossible to ever have children.
- Hysterectomy is not carried out as a standard sterilisation procedure but in response to a number of factors that pose a risk to the woman's health.

The procedure

- Sterilisation involves cutting, clipping, or constricting the fallopian tubes so that sperm cannot reach the egg.
- The surgery is usually performed under general anaesthetic and the woman is likely to have to stay in hospital for a night.
- After the operation, there's a small chance that conception could still occur, depending on the stage in the menstrual cycle. For this reason it's best to use a barrier contraceptive until the first period after sterilisation.

Pros and cons

- Female sterilisation is generally regarded as very effective at preventing pregnancy. But like all operations, there are occasional failures.
- Sterilisation does not affect the quality of a woman's sex life or her sex drive.
- Some women report heavier periods after being sterilised, though it's not known why.
- Sterilisation is not the answer to a rocky relationship. It will only boost your sex life if your relationship is already good by removing anxieties about pregnancy.

Sexual health

Sexually-transmitted diseases can be painful, health-threatening, and even fatal. And with some people unaware that they're even carrying an infection, be sure not to let one night of passion become a killer.

Safer sex facts

Taking precautions with sex is not just sensible, it can be a matter of life or death. The key is to avoid activities involving the exchange of bodily fluids. Sexually-transmitted diseases are transferred from one person to another via semen, blood, or vaginal secretions. When starting a new sexual relationship, use condoms for at least the first few months. You and your partner should then get checked by a doctor and, if you're both given the all-clear and the relationship is monogamous, you can ditch the condoms if you want to.

Best ways to play it safe

1. **Always wear a lubricated condom** When used correctly it forms a physical barrier blocking the exchange of genital fluids between partners.
2. **Spermicides** If used with condoms, spermicides can help kill the HIV virus.
3. **Only use water-based lubricants** Baby oil and other oil-based products can seriously weaken rubber condoms.
4. **Avoid anal sex** The rectal tissues are easily torn, providing an easy route for the transfer of infection.
5. **Think carefully before giving oral sex to a new partner** If you wouldn't find it too embarrassing, you can buy latex sheets, called dental dams, from chemist shops to lay over the woman's vagina.
6. **Infections** They can be passed on via sex toys.
7. **A new partner** Don't rely on someone looking healthy.
8. **Many partners** The more you have, the greater the risk.

Sex and your general health

- **Alcohol** Heavy drinking dents sexual performance. Too many beers can make it difficult to get an erection and limit the production of the male sex hormone testosterone. It also affects libido. About half of all alcoholics have low sex drives.
- **Diet** If you and your partner are aiming for conception, keep up your intake of vitamins and minerals as these play a key role in sperm production. In any case, a balanced diet is fundamental to your general well being.
- **Genital hygiene** It's important to keep your penis and scrotum clean, as failure to do so can be a prompt for some genital cancers. Uncircumcised men should wash under the foreskin every day, using soap or just water to clean away any smegma. Wash around the anus daily.
- **Illnesses** Long-term illnesses, such as diabetes, arthritis, multiple sclerosis, and heart disease can affect sexual activity. But with a supportive partner, sufferers can still enjoy sexual intercourse or mutual masturbation.
- **Medication** A number of medications for hypertension, angina, and other health problems can impair sexual performance.
- **Smoking** It can damage fertility by reducing the sperm production and contributing to a higher proportion of damaged sperm. You know you want to, so stop.
- **Stress** Feeling seriously stressed can have a big impact on your sex drive, and consequently on your relationship. Some men find that although their ability to gain an erection is not affected, the quality of their orgasms is weakened by the fact that they are not truly relaxed. If you are stressed, it's important to separate sources of stress, such as pressure at work, from the bedroom.
- **Underwear** Your choice of underwear can affect your health. It's believed that tight-fitting briefs can reduce a man's sperm count. The material is also important. Underwear made from natural fibres, such as cotton and silk, absorb sweat whereas synthetic materials, like nylon and polyester, don't allow your body to "breathe", prompting a build-up of bacteria in the sweat in the genital area.

DISEASE	HOW ACQUIRED	SYMPTOMS
Chlamydia (bacterial)	Mostly transferred by vaginal or anal intercourse	Stinging; watery discharge; swollen balls; pain peeing
Genital herpes (viral)	Infection spread by contact with an infected area, though there may be no visible signs	Small, itchy blisters around the genitals, similar to cold sores affecting mouths
Gonorrhea (bacterial)	Infection of urethra, rectum, mouth, or throat; passed on by vaginal, anal, or oral sex	Severe pain during urination; yellow discharges from the penis
Hepatitis B and C (viral)	Exchanged via infected blood, semen, vaginal secretions, and saliva	In a third of cases: inflamed liver leading to fever, vomiting, diarrhoea, headaches etc.
HIV/Aids (viral)	Passed on by exposure to contaminated blood	Sufferers of full-blown Aids experience a complete immune system breakdown
Genital warts (human papilloma viral)	Infection through vaginal, anal, or oral sex	Sometimes none, but men tend to develop genital warts around the tip of the penis
Syphilis (bacterial)	Infection through vaginal, anal, or oral sex	Painless ulcer, usually on the penis; rash on the feet or mouth

A guide to common sexually-transmitted diseases

TREATMENT	COMPLICATIONS
Antibiotics, such as erythromycin and tetracycline	If untreated: testicular infection; epididymitis; possible infertility
There's no known cure for herpes; medication can minimise symptoms in severe cases	Open sores can increase the chances of HIV infection
Penicillin cures most cases of gonorrhea	If untreated can lead to infertility and infections of the heart valves, joints, and brain
No cure but both usually clear up on their own within two months. Hep. B is potentially fatal, but a vaccine is available	Advanced symptoms include dark urine, pain in the abdomen, and a yellowing of the skin
Antiviral drugs can slow the development of the HIV infection into Aids	HIV infection resulting from Aids is eventually fatal
No cure for the virus that causes warts, but a doctor can remove them	Complications if not removed: cancers of the penis, anus (and cervix in your partner)
Penicillin will arrest the disease in its early stages, but it won't reverse existing damage	Appalling effects on the brain, heart, joints, and eyes in later stages; possibly fatal

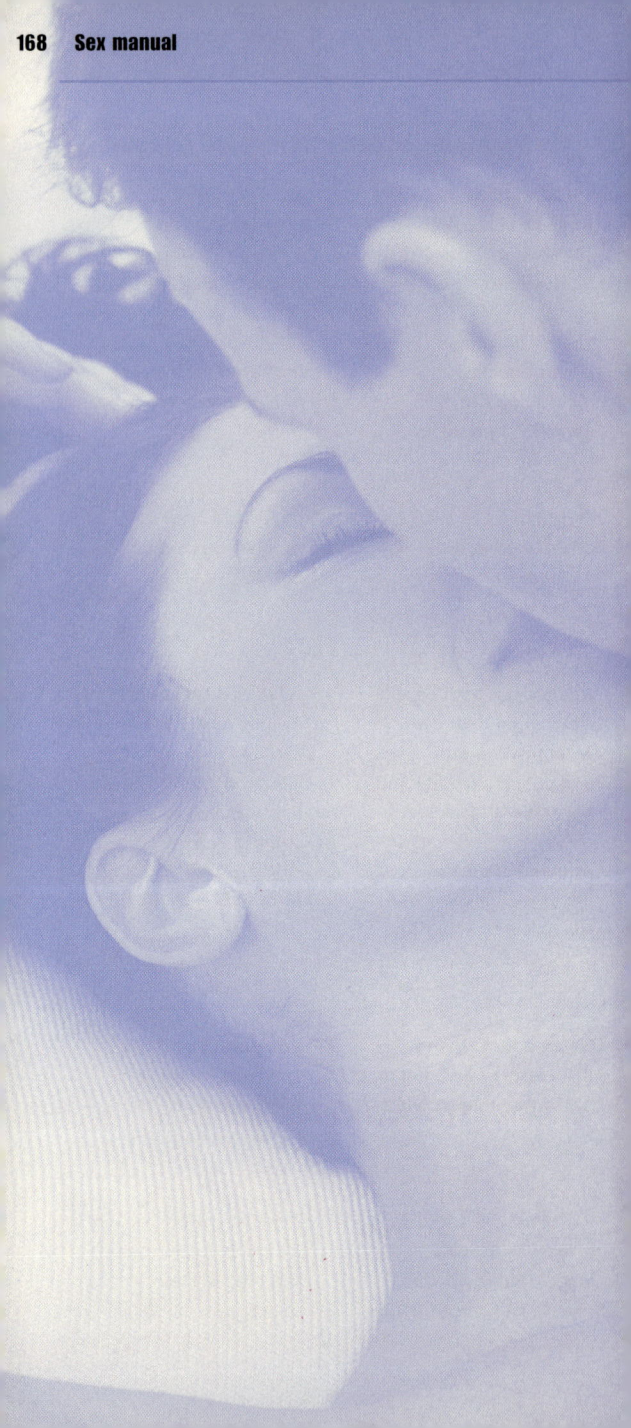

Sex manual

Creative lovemaking
Missionary variations
Basic positions
Face-to-face positions
Rear-entry positions
Advanced positions
Athletic positions

Creative lovemaking

You might wonder what more there is to sex than doing what comes naturally. It depends on your imagination and, with a little creativity, every night can be fireworks night.

Keeping sex alive

- Sex forms such an important bond between partners that when it declines or stagnates, the whole relationship can suffer. One of the biggest dangers of long-term relationships is that sex can easily become dull and routine.
- This is often because you end up using just two or three positions that you've found work best for you both.
- At such times, men's thoughts can stray to the idea of having an affair. The attraction is usually just the novelty of having sex with someone unfamiliar, but it's a cop-out.
- The real solution is to keep sex alive with your partner by trying new positions, feeding off each others' imaginations, and finding out new things about yourselves.

The Kama Sutra

- This ancient Hindu text was written about 2000 years ago by Vatsyayana. Meaning "Aphorisms of Love", the manual shows that desires to add variety to sex are not new.
- In truth, many of the unusual and varied lovemaking positions can only be contemplated by the most supple and gymnastic of lovers, but it's still a good source of inspiration and excitement.

Modern sex manuals

- Today's sex manuals offer many more realistic suggestions. The following pages give an outline of the most popular sex positions, but dedicated sex manuals show a wider range.
- Perhaps the most successful sex manual of the last few decades has been *The Joy of Sex* by Alex Comfort. It broke new ground with its practical and explicit approach to enhancing sex and set a very popular trend.

Positions to suit the person

• Sex can be quite athletic and many positions require flexibility and strength. It's a good idea to try lots of positions to see which best suit the capabilities of you and your partner.
• Men who are overweight, for example, may find that they need to work harder to avoid squashing their partner in some positions, and if you have a bad back, standing sex in which you fully support your partner's weight may cause a slipped disc. Recognise your limitations and work around them.

Start experimenting

• Try some of the following more unusual positions (see p.178–183). If at first they don't seem easy, don't give up.
• Try varying them slightly until they become more enjoyable. Sex is great when it's spontaneous and lustful, but it can be just as enjoyable when it's carefully planned. So if you need to shift a mattress or set up some pillows, do so.
• Recognise that some positions provide significantly more stimulation for one partner than the other, so take it in turns to perform each of your favoured positions.

Top venues for exciting sex

• If you haven't yet moved out of the bedroom, try the bathroom or the shower.
• The stairs can be a good place to get in step with some more interesting sex.
• Sex in the garden can be bloomin' marvellous when the weather permits it – but make sure your neighbours don't get to see your root vegetable.
• Why not try getting her motor running in the car? It might bring back some fond teenage memories.
• What about getting your oats in a country field?
• Railway carriages have a certain coupling attraction.
• And sex in the sea can give you waves of pleasure.
Note: While having sex outdoors can add a frisson of excitement with the prospect of being caught, be aware that you could be arrested for breaking the law.

Missionary variations

The basic missionary position is probably the simplest of all positions. The woman lies on her back with her legs apart and the man lies on top with his legs inside hers. The position is wonderfully intimate as it allows the lovers to kiss and look into one another's eyes. The only disadvantage is that the woman may have little control over the proceedings. She can, however, vary the position by moving her pelvis up and down, opening her legs wider, or wrapping them around her partner.

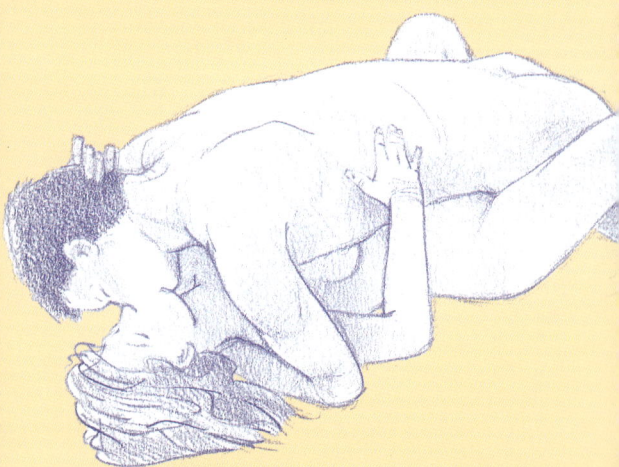

CLASSIC MISSIONARY
This most basic of positions is maligned as much for the monotonous regularity with which many couples practise it as for anything intrinsically boring about the position itself. It allows great face-to-face intimacy, deep penetration, and easy thrusting. The man dominates the action. Tip: Support your weight on your elbows and allow your partner some room to move.

Missionary variations

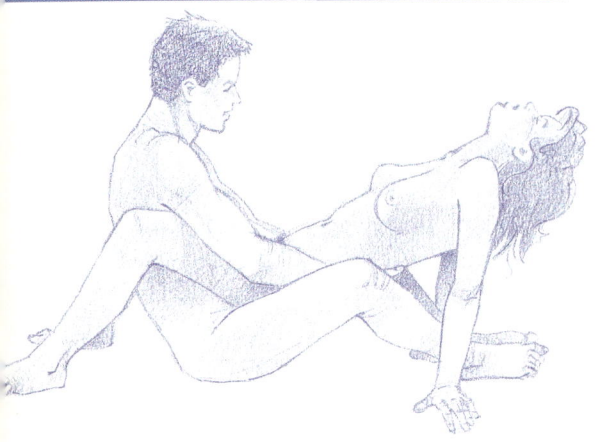

SEATED MISSIONARY

This variation on the missionary position isn't as strenuous for the man or as weighty on the woman. Thrusting isn't quite as easy but that gives you more control over orgasm. Many couples find they can be joyously locked in this position for considerable lengths of time.

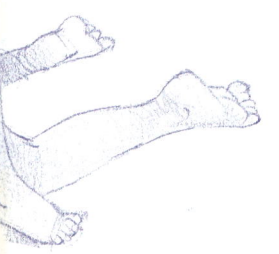

REVERSE MISSIONARY

This is a good position for men who want to delay their orgasm. It also suits couples where the man's weight and size dwarfs his partner's. The woman can also put her legs inside the man's or rest both on top enabling her to rub her clitoris directly against the man's body.

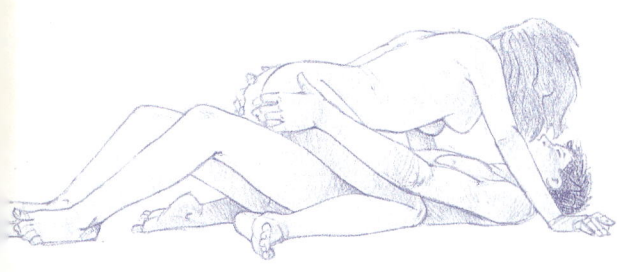

Basic positions

Rear-entry is generally more popular with men than with women, partly because of its animalistic, carnal overtones. The spoons position is an intimate and effortless position, perfect for long, loving, relaxing sex. The many advantages of the woman astride position is the view the man has of his lover's body, particularly her breasts. The clitoris can be stimulated by either the man or the women.

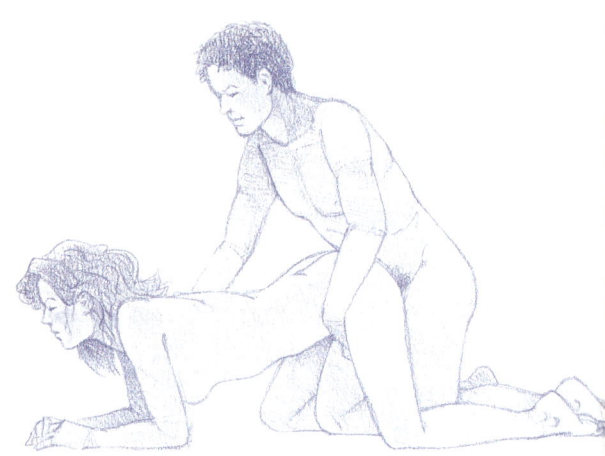

CLASSIC REAR ENTRY
A major advantage of this position is that it allows deep vaginal penetration at an angle that brings the penis into direct contact with the hotly-debated G-spot. A potential disadvantage, however, is that it offers little in the way of clitoral stimulation – although your hands can easily remedy this drawback.

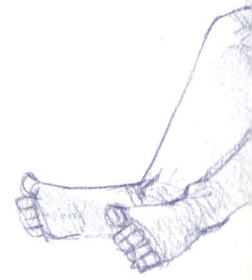

Basic positions 175

SPOONS

Penetration can be a bit tricky to maintain but slight shifts in position can improve the angle. Thrusting isn't easy in the spoons position, but athleticism isn't the point here. Spooning is ideal for pregnant women or overweight men.

WOMAN ASTRIDE

The woman has control over the angle and depth of penetration. She can also control the rhythm and pace of the movement. The man can simply relax. This position helps the man control his orgasm. The woman can take some of her weight off her partner by leaning back and supporting herself on his thighs.

Face-to-face positions

Positions in which the partners are facing one another are among the most romantic. Face-to-face sex is often more popular with women because the animalistic associations of rear-entry sex and the carnal fervour that it instills in some men are absent. All these positions allow for eye contact and, in the case of the standing and facing spoons positions, prolonged kissing. The woman-on-top leaning back position is one of the best for clitoral stimulation – the man has no excuses for not being able to make contact with the love bud.

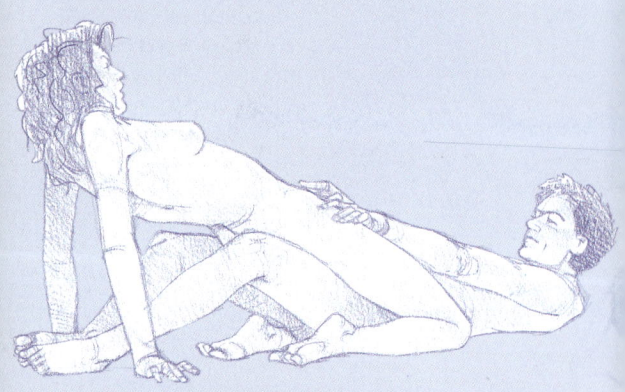

WOMAN-ON-TOP, LEANING BACK
This variation on the woman-astride position – all she has to do is lean back – affords the man superb manual access to her clitoris. He can easily rise up on his elbows for a better view of the situation. There's a similar variation to this: the woman-on-top, facing-away position. In this case she's lying with her back on the man's chest. He can't touch her clitoris so easily, but it puts her breasts within easy reach.

Face-to-face positions

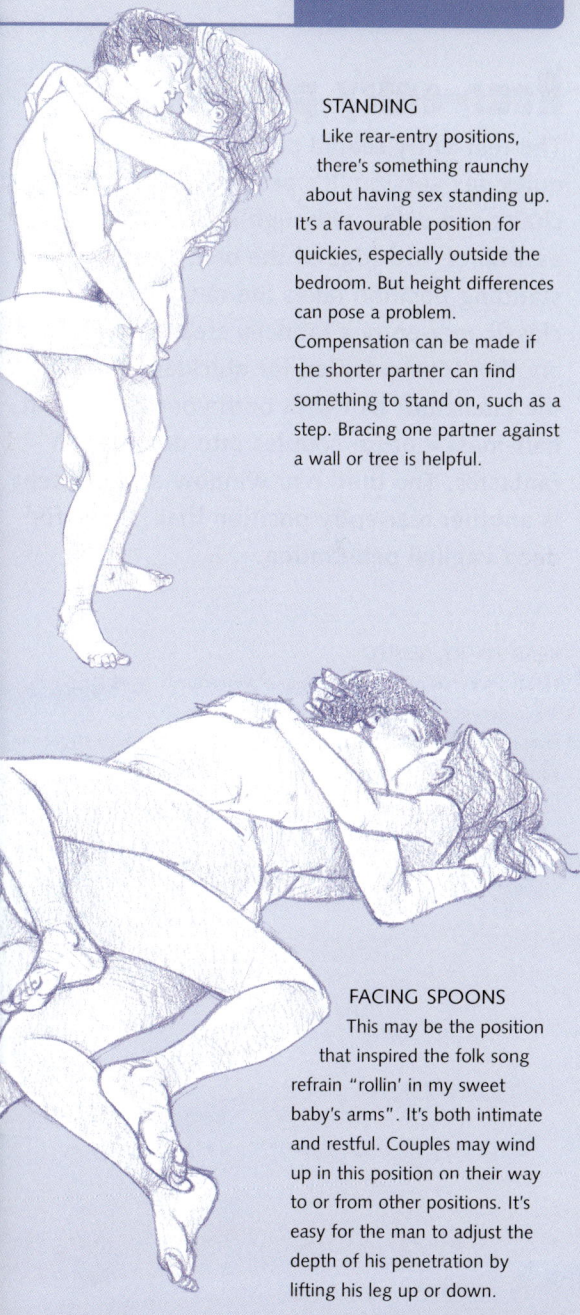

STANDING
Like rear-entry positions, there's something raunchy about having sex standing up. It's a favourable position for quickies, especially outside the bedroom. But height differences can pose a problem. Compensation can be made if the shorter partner can find something to stand on, such as a step. Bracing one partner against a wall or tree is helpful.

FACING SPOONS
This may be the position that inspired the folk song refrain "rollin' in my sweet baby's arms". It's both intimate and restful. Couples may wind up in this position on their way to or from other positions. It's easy for the man to adjust the depth of his penetration by lifting his leg up or down.

Rear-entry positions

The rear-entry seated position is perfect for a quick sex session. It's probably best suited for chairs and sofas, although it can be done just as well on the edge of the bed. The rear-entry standing position takes the rawness of the classic rear-entry a raunchy step further. It's another ideal position for quickies – try it in the kitchen or hall with both your knickers at half-mast – or for couples into domination fantasies. The third rear window arrangement is another rear-entry position that makes for deep vaginal penetration.

REAR-ENTRY, SEATED

The woman has plenty of freedom of movement, assuming her legs are in decent shape. The man can relax, although he can gain some leverage for thrusting by putting his weight on his hands. Each partner can simultaneously stimulate the other's erogenous zones by hand.

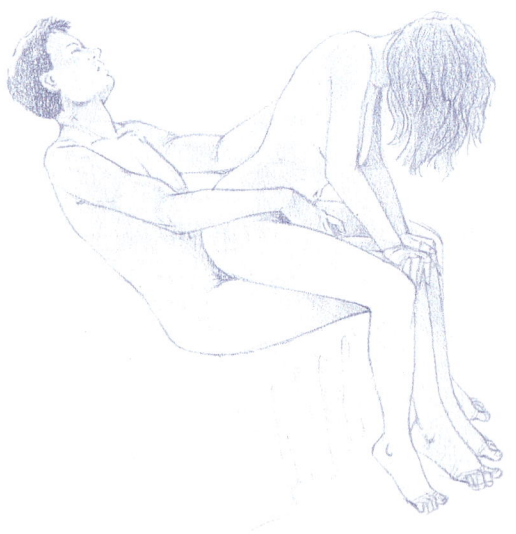

Rear-entry positions

REAR-ENTRY, STANDING
Big differences in height can be overcome by having the shorter partner stand on a pile of sex manuals or other weighty tomes. You might also try this on a flight of stairs, although having a banister to hold onto would be a good idea.

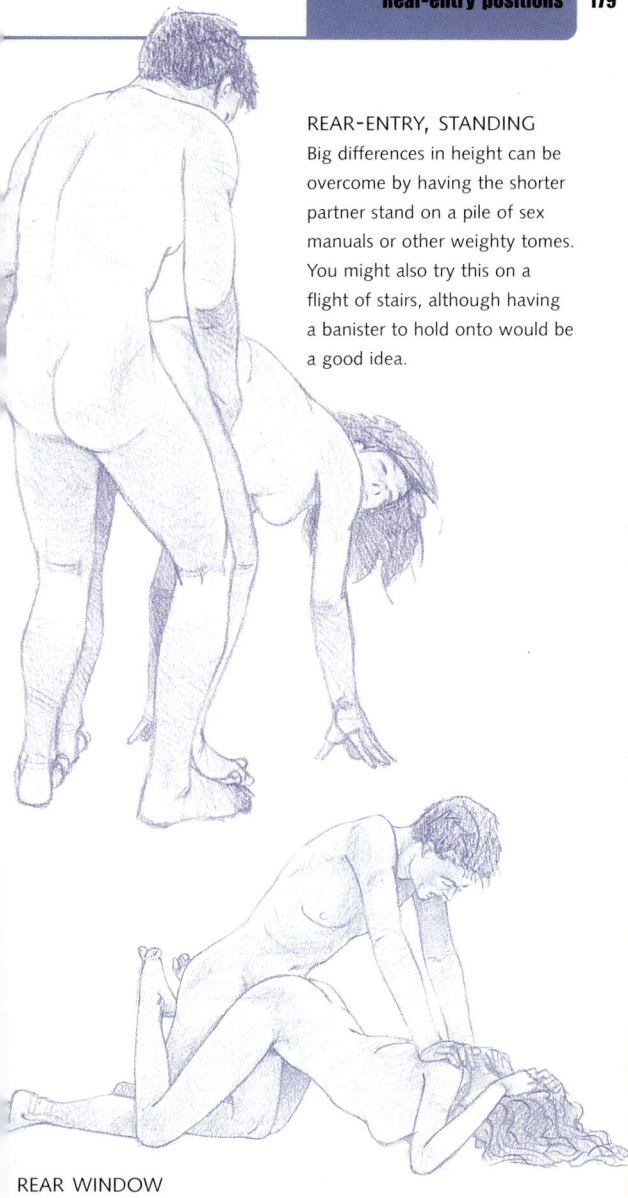

REAR WINDOW
The woman kneels on the bed, supported on her elbows with hands clasped behind her head. The man then kneels behind and positions himself to enter her. Contact is made particularly raunchy when she hooks her legs around his and pulls him towards her.

Advanced positions

With the woman astride and facing away, each partner has a certain degree of freedom to indulge in sexual fantasy, although the man might he happy just to gaze at his partner's backside. The X position is ideal for couples who want a session of slow, leisurely sex. The knees-to-chest position is sometimes called the "Rutting Deer". It's a more athletic variation on the standard missionary position, and allows for the deepest possible penetration of the vagina.

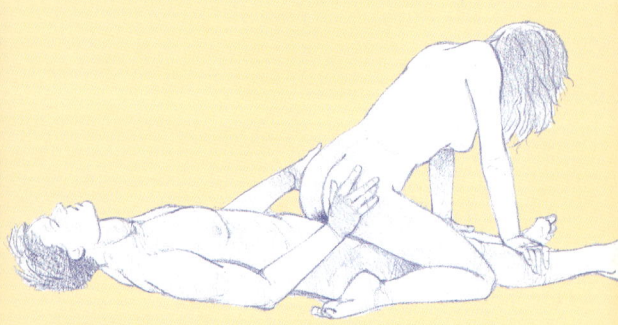

WOMAN ASTRIDE, FACING AWAY
She can caress her partner's testicles and her own clitoris while he rubs her shoulders and buttocks, perhaps with some erotic massage oil. The main advantage of this position for the woman is the depth of penetration and also the freedom of movement it affords. For even greater mobility, the woman can rise up in a squat.

KNEES-TO-CHEST

Getting into this position isn't as tricky as it might look. Start in the woman-astride position, then lean back, adjust your legs into a scissors position and grasp one another's hands. But go carefully – this position can force the penis down at an angle it's not used to.

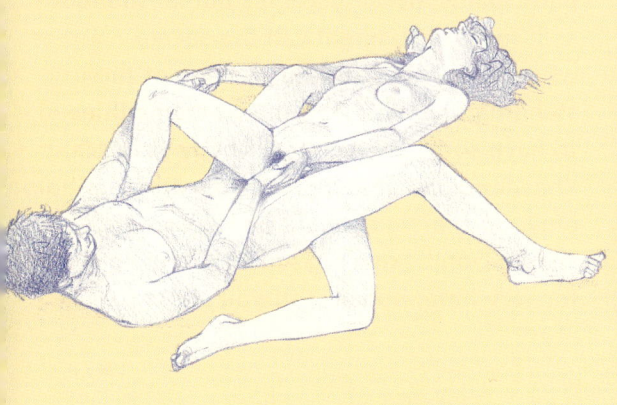

THE X POSITION

The penetration in this position is so deep, it's recommended for couples who wish to conceive. The man's penis is positioned right at the opening of the cervix when he ejaculates. The woman lifts her knees up to her chest, hooking them over the man's shoulders. The man is easily able to press his pubic bone against the clitoris.

Athletic positions

Kneeling positions, such as the reverse missionary squat, combine intimacy with a degree of athleticism, although once both participants are in place, it's not as strenuous as it looks. You might call the seated wheelbarrow the amateur version of the standing one, although the woman will need to have some serious upper-body strength. The standing variation is for the athletic only: both of you should be in good shape. Don't expect to hold the position for very long, however fit you are.

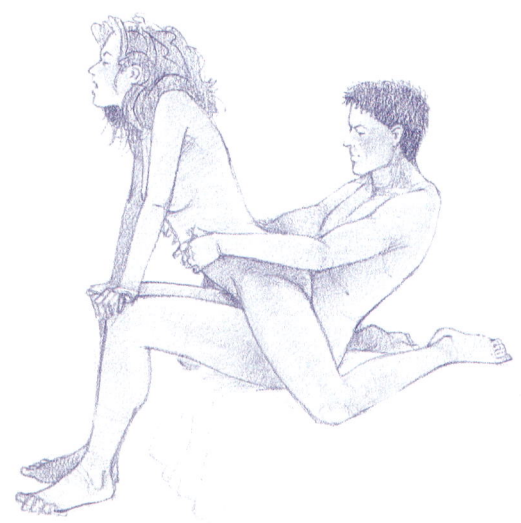

SEATED WHEELBARROW

This is not a position you should expect to stay in for a very long time, but it's a fun alternative that offers an unusual angle of entry – not to mention a nice view of her backside.

Athletic positions

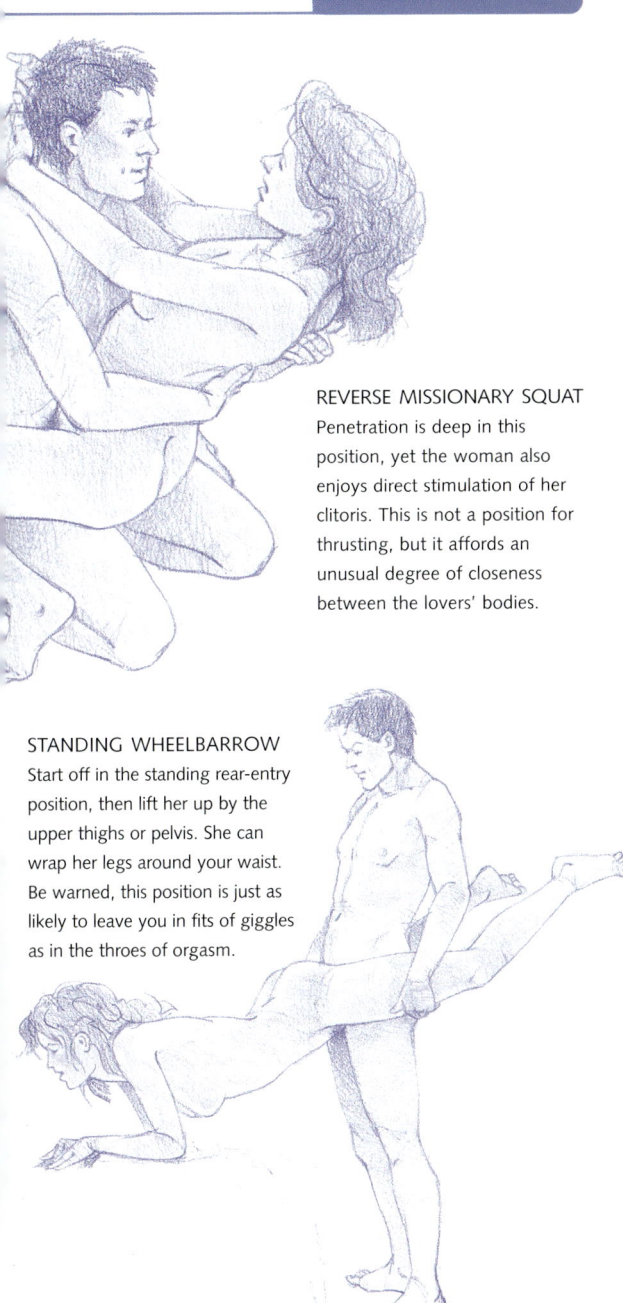

REVERSE MISSIONARY SQUAT
Penetration is deep in this position, yet the woman also enjoys direct stimulation of her clitoris. This is not a position for thrusting, but it affords an unusual degree of closeness between the lovers' bodies.

STANDING WHEELBARROW
Start off in the standing rear-entry position, then lift her up by the upper thighs or pelvis. She can wrap her legs around your waist. Be warned, this position is just as likely to leave you in fits of giggles as in the throes of orgasm.

Index

A
abdomen, massage, 124
Abraham Lincoln beards, 48
aches and pains, 24
acne, 37, 39, 46, 81
additives, food, 79
aerobic exercise, 20, 74
affairs, 170
afterplay, 137
aftershave, 46, 47, 50
Agassi, André, 48
ageing, 20–1
 impotency, 154
AIDS, 19, 131, 140, 166–7
aids, sexual, 146–7, 164
alcohol, 19, 76–7
 benefits of, 76
 binge drinking, 15
 hangover cures, 77
 and healthy sperm, 133
 and heart disease, 19
 and ill-health, 61, 76
 and impotence, 150
 and insomnia, 23
 safe limits, 77
 and sex, 165
 and skin, 37
 and weight gain, 75
allergies, 79, 81
alpha hydroxy acids (AHAs), 37
amino acids, 41, 62
anal intercourse, 141, 164
anger, 85
angina, 165
animal genitalia, aphrodisiacs, 153
anniversaries, 93
antioxidants, 21, 64, 81
antiperspirants, 51
anus:
 anal intercourse, 141, 164
 digestive system, 69
aphrodisiacs, 152–3
apocrine glands, 50
armpits, body odour, 50
arms:
 body language, 87
 massage, 124
aromatherapy massage, 122
arousal, 130, 134
arteries:
 overweight and, 72
 problems, 21, 72, 154
arthritis, 81, 165
asparagus, as aphrodisiac, 153
aspirin, 77
athletic positions, intercourse, 182–3

B
back:
 back pain, 24
 massage, 124
bacteria:
 bad breath, 52
 body odour, 50, 51
 sexually transmitted diseases, 166–7
 tooth decay, 54
bad breath, 52
baking soda, mouthwashes, 53
balding, 44–5, 81
barbers, 43
barrier methods, contraception, 158–9
baths, 33, 51
beards, 48–9
 shaving, 46–7
Beatnik beards, 48
bedrooms, 23
beer, 19, 77
benzoyl peroxide, 39
best friend status, 91
beta-carotene, 21, 65
Billings method, contraception, 160
binge drinking, 15
biotin, 65
birthdays, 93
biting nails, 57
blackened nails, 57
blackheads, 36
bladder, 132
bleaching hair, 43, 49
blindfolds, bondage, 144
blood pressure see high blood pressure
blood sugar levels, 61
body hair, 49, 110
body language, 86–7
body odour, 50–1
body rubbing, 141
bondage, 144
bones, ageing, 20
boxer shorts, 148
brain:
 ageing, 20
 alcohol and, 76
 diet and, 27
 during sex, 131
 endorphins, 32
 mental abilities, 15, 21
 sleep, 22
breakfast, 61
breaking up, 96
breasts:
 arousal, 134
 outercourse, 141
 puberty, 110
breathing, relaxation, 32, 33
briefs, 148, 165
British Medical Association, 77
bruises, 57
burns, 38
Buss, David, 91

C
caffeine, 18
calcium, 66, 80
calluses, on feet, 37
calories, 71, 74, 75
cancer:
 colon cancer, 61, 72
 free radicals and, 21
 genital cancer, 165
 liver cancer, 76
 lung cancer, 18
 prostate cancer, 72
 smoking and, 18

cap, contraceptive, 159
carbohydrates, 60, 61
   sources of, 63
   and stress, 27
   uses, 62
   and weight loss, 74
cataracts, 21
Catholic church, 112, 160
Caverject, 151, 155
celery seeds, as aphrodisiac, 153
cervical cap, contraceptive, 159
chatting-up, 100–1
chest hair, 49
chewing gum, 57
Chinese rings, 146
chlamydia, 166–7
chloride, 66
cholesterol, 72
   alcohol and, 76
   fibre and, 61
   lowering levels of, 74
   sources of, 60
cigarettes see smoking
circulatory problems, impotence, 150
cirrhosis, 76
climax see orgasm
clitoris, 128
   arousal, 130, 134
   clitoral stimulators, 147
   oral sex, 126, 127
   orgasm, 117, 128, 135
clothes, 102–5
   buying, 103
   colour, 102
   fetish clothes, 145
   shirts, 104–5
   suits, 104–5
   underwear, 148–9, 165
clubs, sado-masochism, 145
cock rings, 147
coffee, 18, 23
coil, contraceptive, 157
cold sores, 127
colitis, 81
collagen, 38
colognes, 50
colon:
   cancer, 61, 72
   digestion, 69
colour:
   clothes, 102
   hair dyes, 43
Comfort, Alex, 170
commitment, 94
communication, 8–9, 84–9, 95
compatibility, 95
compliments, 101
compromises, 95
computers:
   computerised contraception, 161
   and skin disorders, 24
condoms, 19, 158–9
   anal intercourse, 141
   putting on, 159
   safe sex, 164
   sex toys, 146
   types, 158
conflicts, 94

contraception, 115, 140, 156–63
control, 14–15
   work environment, 29
copper, 80
cosmetics, 7, 36
costumes, sexual fantasies, 143
counsellors, 88, 116
cramps, 67
credit cards, 27
Crohn's disease, 81
crow's feet, 37
crying, 27, 67
cunnilingus, 126–7
cuticles, 56
cuts and grazes, 38
cycling, 20, 27, 74, 75

D

dairy products, 63, 68
dandruff, 40, 41, 49
dating, 99–101
   finding a date, 96–7
   first moves, 100–1
   new relationships, 106–7
death, alcohol and, 76
dehydration, 67, 77
delegation, 16, 31
dental care, 15, 53–5
dental dams, 164
dentine, teeth, 54
deodorants, 51
depilatories, 49
depression, 154
dermatitis, 39
dermis, 36, 38
desserts, 75
diabetes, 150, 154, 165
diet, 8, 15, 59–71
   and acne, 39
   and ageing, 20
   alcohol, 76–7
   aphrodisiacs, 152
   bad breath, 52
   and body odour, 51
   fibre, 67
   food pyramid, 60, 68
   food supplements, 80–1
   and hair, 41
   and healthy sperm, 133
   and insomnia, 23
   major food groups, 62–3
   menu planning guide, 70–1
   minerals, 66
   nail care, 57
   organic food, 78–9
   and sex, 165
   and sleep, 61
   and stress, 27
   vitamins, 64–5
dieting, 61, 75
digestive system, 69
   fibre and, 67
   stress and, 24
dihydrotestosterone, 44
dildos, 127, 146, 147
diseases see sexually transmitted diseases
displacement activity, body language, 87

divorce, 151
doctors, 14
drinking see alcohol
drugs:
  and hair regrowth, 45
  and sex, 165
  sex drive drugs, 151, 155
  sleep-inducing, 23
dry skin, 37
dutch cap, 159
dyes, hair, 43

E
ear hair, 49
eczema, 37, 39, 81
eggs:
  female sterilisation, 163
  menstrual cycle, 161
ejaculation, 138
  fellatio, 129
  masturbation, 112
  multiple orgasm, 139
  orgasm, 130, 132–3
elastin, 20
electric beard trimmers, 49
electric shavers, 46
electric toothbrushes, 54
electrolysis, hair removal, 49
Elvis Presley beards, 48
emails, 30
emotions:
  controlling, 85
  recognising, 14
  work environment, 29
enamel, teeth, 54
endorphins, 32
energy, diet and, 62
enzymes, 69, 81
epidermis, 36, 38
erections, 111, 130
  Caverject, 151
  impotence, 150, 154–5
  "outercourse", 140
  Viagra, 151
  see also ejaculation
erogenous zones, 119, 121, 135
essential oils, 120, 122, 123
evening primrose oil, 81
exercise, 15, 71
  aerobic exercise, 74
  and ageing, 20
  and insomnia, 23
  and stress, 27
  stretching exercises, 32, 33
  and weight gain, 71, 73, 74, 75
exfoliation, 36
eye contact, body language, 86, 89,100
eyes:
  ageing, 20
  crow's feet, 37

F
face-to-face positions, intercourse, 176–7
facial scrubs, 36
facing spoons position, intercourse, 177
faeces, 69

fallopian tubes, 163
fantasies, sexual, 93, 113, 121, 142–3
fasting, 61
fatigue, 22
fats, 60, 61
  food pyramid, 68
  losing weight, 74, 75
  slowing down ageing, 20
  sources of, 63
  uses, 62
  see also cholesterol
feelings see emotions
feet:
  massage, 124
  skin care, 37
  smelly feet, 51
fellatio, 129
female genitals, 128
female orgasm, 134–5
female sterilisation, 163
feminism, 91
fetish clothes, 145
fibre, in diet, 60, 61, 67
financial problems, 27
fingernails see nails
first aid, skin, 38
fish oils, 81
flossing teeth, 15, 53
flowers, 93, 120
fluff inspection, body language, 87
folic acid, 65
food see diet
food additives, 79
food pyramid, 60, 68
food supplements, 80–1
football, 74
foreplay, 90, 118–21
  dirty phone calls, 120
  fantasies, 121
  kissing, 121
  oral sex, 126, 129
foreskin, 111, 165
forgiveness, 95
free radicals, 21, 81
Freud, Sigmund, 117
friends, 91, 106
fruit, 60, 63
  antioxidants, 21
  food pyramid, 68
  fruit juice, 77
  and skin, 37
  slowing down ageing, 20
fungal problems, nails, 57

G
G-spot, 135
gallbladder, 69
games, sexual, 142–3
gamma linolenic acid, 81
garlic, 81
gels, hair styling, 40, 41
genetically modified (GM) food, 78
genetics, and weight gain, 73
genital herpes, 166–7
genital warts, 166–7
genitals:
  body odour, 50

female, 128
  oral sex, 126–7
  see also penis; vagina
gifts, 93
gingivitis, 52
ginseng:
  as aphrodisiac, 153
  as supplement, 81
glans, penis, 111
glucose, 62
goals, 16
goatee beards, 48
gonorrhea, 127, 166–7
grains, 20, 21, 60, 63, 68
Gray, John, 84
grey hair, 43
grinding teeth, 55
gum disease, 52, 54

H
hair, 40–9
  ageing, 20
  beards, 48–9
  body hair, 49, 110
  and diet, 41
  dyes, 43
  ear hair, 49
  grey hair, 43
  hair care, 40–1
  hair loss, 44–5
  ingrown hairs, 47
  nose hair, 49
  pubic hair, 110
  replacement treatments, 45
  shaving, 46–7
  shaving head, 45
  styles, 42
  stylists, 43
hair follicles, 38
  acne, 39
  electrolysis, 49
  hair loss, 44
  ingrown hairs, 47
hairpieces, 44
hands:
  body language, 87
  massage, 124
  nails, 56–7
handshakes, 87
hangnails, 57
hangover cures, 77
head rub, 33
headaches, 24, 81, 122
health, sexual, 164–7
heart, ageing, 20
heart attacks, 72
heart disease:
  alcohol and, 19, 76
  cholesterol and, 72
  diet and, 60
  and impotency, 154
  overweight and, 15
  and sex, 165
  stress and, 24
heartburn, 24, 61
hepatitis, 141, 166–7
herpes, genital, 166–7
high blood pressure:
  alcohol and, 76
  overweight and, 15, 72
  stress and, 24, 26
Hite, Shere, 117
HIV, 19, 141, 164, 166–7
holidays, 12, 31
honesty, 95, 100
hormones:
  contraceptive pill, 156, 157
  in puberty, 110
  and stress, 27
  see also testosterone
human papilloma virus, 166–7
humour, 32, 101
hydrochloric acid, 69
hygiene:
  genital, 165
  oral hygiene, 52–5
  personal hygiene, 50–1
hygienists, dental, 53
hymen, 115
hysterectomy, 163

I
illness, and sex, 165
immune system, 19, 81
implants, penile, 155
impotence, 81, 112, 154–5
indigestion, 61
individuality, 95
ingrown hairs, 47
insomnia, 23, 61
intercourse see sex
intestines, digestion, 69
intrauterine device (IUD), 157
iron, 80
irritable bowel syndrome, 24

J
jackets, 103, 104–5
Jews, 112
jogging, 74
Johnson, Virginia, 117

K
Kama Sutra, 152, 170
Kegel exercises, 139
keratin, 44
kidneys, ageing, 20
Kilmer, Val, 48
Kinsey, Alfred, 117
kissing, 121
knees-to-chest position, intercourse, 181

L
labia, 128
  arousal, 130, 134
  oral sex, 126
laughter, 32, 33, 101
leather clothing, bondage, 144
leather shoes, 51
lecithin, 21, 81
legs, massage, 124
leisure, 16, 27, 31
libido, 165
lifestyle, changing, 12–13
lighting, 120
listening, 88–9

liver:
  alcohol and, 76
  cancer, 76
  cholesterol, 72
  digestion, 69
love, 12, 94–5, 106, 107
love balls, 147
lovemaking see sex
lubricants, 146
  anal intercourse, 141
  masturbation, 113
  safe sex, 164
lunches, 75
lung cancer, 18
lymph system, 69

M

magnesium, 66, 80
malaria, anti-malarial tablets, 41
male-pattern baldness, 44
male pill, 157
marriage, 12
masks, sexual fantasies, 143
masochism, 145
massage, 122–5
massage oils, 123, 146
Masters, William, 117
masturbation, 112–13, 131
  body rubbing, 141
  clitoris, 117, 135
  sensate focusing, 155
meat, 62, 63
meditation, 32, 33
melanin, hair colour, 43
memory:
  ageing, 21
  sleep and, 22
menstruation, 140, 161
mental abilities, 15, 21
mental attitudes, 15, 17
menu planning guide, 70–1
metabolic rate, 20, 71, 72, 75
minerals, 60, 61, 66, 71
  food supplements, 80
  and hair, 41
Minoxidil, 45
missionary positions, intercourse, 172–3, 180–1
moisturisers, 36, 37, 38
  after shaving, 46
  nail care, 56
money problems, 27
monosodium glutamate, 79
monounsaturated oils, 63
morning-after contraceptive pill, 156
mousse, hair styling, 40, 41
moustaches, 48
mouth:
  digestion, 69
  oral hygiene, 52–5
mouthwashes, 53
multiple orgasms, 138–9
multiple sclerosis, 165
muscles:
  aerobic exercise, 74
  ageing, 20
  cramps, 67
  exercise, 15
  massage, 122
  protein and, 62
  relaxation, 33
MUSE technique, impotency, 155

N

nails, 56–7
  diet and, 41
  grooming, 56
  problems, 57
naps, 23, 27
natural methods, contraception, 160–1
neck, massage, 124
neck scratching, body language, 87
negative thoughts, 33
"new man" culture, 91
niacin, 64
nicks, shaving, 47
nicotine skin patches, 18
nipples, arousal, 134
"No", saying, 16
nose hair, 49
nutrition see diet

O

obesity see overweight
oils:
  essential, 120, 122, 123
  fish, 81
  massage, 123, 146
oily skin, 37, 39
oral hygiene, 52–5
oral sex, 126–9, 140, 164
organic food, 78–9
organs, ageing, 20
orgasm, 117, 130
  delaying, 131
  female, 128, 134–5
  foreplay, 118
  intensifying, 136–7
  male, 132–3
  multiple orgasms, 138–9
  oral sex, 126
  vibrators, 147
outercourse, 140–1
overweight, 15, 72–5
  exercise and, 71, 73, 74, 75
  personal hygiene and, 51
Ovid, 152
ovulation, 160, 161, 163
oxygen, smoking and, 18
oysters, as aphrodisiac, 153

P

pain, 14
  hangover cures, 77
  sado-masochism, 145
  stress and, 24
pancreas, 69
pantothenic acid, 64
paracetamol, 77
passion, 92–3
penis, 111
  Caverject, 151
  clitoral stimulators, 147
  condoms, 159

fellatio, 129
implants, 155
impotence, 150, 154–5
orgasm, 132
outercourse, 140, 141
puberty, 110
rings, 146, 147
see also erections
percussion, massage, 125
perineum, 113, 141
periodontitis, 52
periods, 140, 161
Persona, contraception, 161
personal hygiene, 50–1
pesticides, 78
petroleum jelly, 57
pheromones, 50
phosphorus, 66
pill, contraceptive, 156, 157
pimples, 39
plant seeds, 63
plaque, 52, 54
plateau, sexual arousal, 130
pollution, 78
polyunsaturated oils, 63
positive thinking, 15, 17
posture:
  aches and pains, 24
  body language, 86
potassium, 66, 80
potency, 150–1
pregnancy, 131, 140
premenstrual tension (PMT), 161
Presley, Elvis, 48
pressing, massage, 125
promotion, 17
Propecia, 45
prostate cancer, 72
prostate gland, 130, 132
proteins, 60, 61
  and ageing, 20
  food pyramid, 68
  and hair, 41
  sources of, 63
  uses, 62
psoriasis, 39, 81
psychology, sexual, 116–17
puberty, 110–11
pubic hair, 110
pubic mound, 128
pubococcygeal (PC) muscles:
  delaying orgasm, 131, 139
  intensifying orgasm, 136
  vaginal orgasm, 135
pulp, teeth, 54
pulse, stress and, 26
PVC clothing, bondage, 144

R

rashes, 24, 39
razors, 46, 47
rear-entry positions, intercourse, 174, 178–9
rear window position, intercourse, 179
rectum, 69
Regaine, 45
relationships, 8, 83–97

best friend status, 91
conflicts, 94
dating, 99–107
finding a date, 96–7
listening, 88–9
love, 94–5
new relationships, 106–7
passion, 92–3
supporting your partner, 90
talking, 84–5
work and, 29
see also sex
relaxation, 32–3
coping with stress, 27
and insomnia, 23
laughter, 32
workaholism, 31
reverse missionary positions, intercourse, 173, 180–1
reverse missionary squat, intercourse, 181
rheumatoid arthritis, 81
rhino horn, as aphrodisiac, 153
rhythm method, contraception, 160
riboflavin, 64
rings, Chinese, 146, 147
romance, 92
rosacea, 39
royal jelly, 81
running, 27

S

sado-masochism (S&M), 145
safe sex, 164
saliva, 52, 69
salt, mouthwashes, 53
saturated fat, 72
  cholesterol levels, 60, 61
  lowering, 74
  sources of, 63
scalp massage, 33
scars, 39
scratching, body language, 87
scrotum, 111, 131
  hygiene, 165
  puberty, 110
seated missionary position, intercourse, 173
sebaceous glands, 38, 39
sebum, 39
selenium, 21, 80
semen, 111
  ejaculation, 130, 132, 138–9
  fellatio, 129
  "wet dreams", 112
sensate focusing, 155
sensual massage, 124
serotonin, 27
sex, 9, 95, 109–67
  aftermath, 107, 137
  alternatives to intercourse, 140–1
  anal sex, 164
  aphrodisiacs, 152–3
  benefits of, 19
  bondage, 144
  contraception, 156–63
  fantasies, 142–3
  foreplay, 90, 118–21

four stages of response, 130
games, 142–3
impotency, 154–5
keeping sex alive, 93
losing virginity, 114–15
making it last, 131
masturbation, 112–13, 131, 135, 141
new relationships, 107
oral sex, 126–9, 140, 164
orgasm, 132–9
passion, 92–3
pheromones, 50
positions, 131, 170, 171, 172–83
potency, 150–1
psychology, 116–17
in puberty, 110
sado-masochism (S&M), 145
sex manual, 169–83
sexual aids, 93, 146–7, 164
sexual health, 164–7
talking and, 85
sex therapy, 116, 140
sexually transmitted diseases, 166–7
anal intercourse, 141
condoms, 19, 164
oral sex, 127
outercourse, 140
safe sex, 164
shampoo, 40, 41, 49
shaving, 46–7
body hair, 49
head, 45
shirts, 102, 104–5, 148
shoes, 103
fungal problems, 57
smelly feet, 51
shoulders:
massage, 124
stretching exercises, 32
showers, 51
sideburns, 48
"69" position, 127
skin:
ageing, 20
ailments, 39
first aid, 38
skin care, 36–7
stress and, 24
structure, 38
skin patches, nicotine, 18
sleep, 15, 22–3
diet and, 61
and stress, 27
smegma, 111, 165
smells, 50–1
smoking, 15
bad breath, 52
and impotence, 150
and insomnia, 23
nail care, 57
quitting, 18, 27
and sex, 165
and skin, 37
snacks, 61
snakes, as aphrodisiac, 153
soap:
antibacterial, 51, 57
deodorant, 51

shaving, 47
washing face, 36, 37
social life, 14, 28
socks, 51, 103, 148
sodium, 66
Soil Association, 79
Soul Patch beards, 48
Spanish fly, 153
spanking, sado-masochism, 145
sperm, 111
alcohol and, 76
contraception, 157
masturbation, 112
orgasm, 130, 132–3
vasectomy, 162
spermicides, 158, 159, 164
spirits, 19
spiritual activities, 33
spoons position, intercourse, 175, 177
sport, 27
stained nails, 57
stained teeth, 54
standing position, intercourse, 177
sterilisation, 162–3
stomach, digestion, 69
Stop 'n' Grow, 57
stress, 7, 24–7
and impotence, 150
reducing, 26–7
and sex, 165
and skin, 37
stretching exercises, 32, 33
strokes:
alcohol and, 76
overweight and, 72
strokes, massage, 125
stubble, 48
sugar, 60, 62, 63, 68
suicide, 76
suits, 102, 103, 104–5
sun, effects on skin, 20, 37
sun screen, 37
sunburn, 38
superoxide dismutase (SOD), 81
supplements, 80–1
supporting your partner, 90
surgery, sterilisation, 162–3
surprises, 93
sweat glands, 36, 38, 50, 51
sweating, 15, 51, 67
swimming, 20, 27, 74
syphilis, 166–7

T
talking, 84–5
foreplay, 119
tartar, 52, 54
teeth:
cleaning, 15, 53, 54–5
decay, 52, 54
grinding, 55
telephone calls, foreplay, 120
television, 23, 30
temper, losing, 85
tennis, 27, 74
testicles, 111
ejaculation, 132

fellatio, 129
orgasm, 131
puberty, 110
testosterone, 111, 151
and ageing, 20
male-pattern baldness, 44
potency, 150
puberty, 110
therapy:
counselling, 88
sex therapy, 116, 140
thiamin, 21, 64
thirst, 67
threesomes, 93
ties, 102
time:
and relationships, 95
time management, 30
tiredness, 22
toenails see nails
tongue:
bad breath, 52
oral sex, 127
toothbrushes, 54
touch, foreplay, 119
trousers, 102, 148
buying, 103
styles, 104–5
truffles, as aphrodisiac, 153
tweezing hairs, 49

U
ulcerative colitis, 81
underwear, 148–9, 165
unsaturated oils, 63
urethra, 111, 128, 132
urine, 67, 111, 132
uterus, 134, 135, 163

V
vacuum therapy, impotency, 155
vagina:
arousal, 130, 134
foreplay, 118
G-spot, 135
love balls, 147
oral sex, 126, 127
virginity, 115
Valentine's day, 93
Vandyke beards, 48
vas deferens, 132, 162
vasectomy, 162
vegan diet, 63
vegetable oils, 63
vegetables, 60, 63
antioxidants, 21
food pyramid, 68
and skin, 37
slowing down ageing, 20
vegetarian diet, 63
Viagra, 151, 155
vibrators, 146, 147
virginity, losing, 114–15
viruses, sexually-transmitted diseases, 166-7
vitamins, 60, 61, 64–5, 71
food supplements, 80
and hair, 41

vitamin A, 21, 65, 80
vitamin B complex, 21, 64–5, 80
vitamin C, 21, 64, 77, 80
vitamin D, 65, 80
vitamin E, 21, 65, 80
vitamin K, 65
vulva, 128
oral sex, 127

W
warts, genital, 166–7
washing:
face, 36, 37
hair, 40, 41
water, drinking, 37, 60, 61, 67, 77
waxing, hair removal, 49
weaving, hair dyes, 43, 45
weight, 72–5
exercise and, 71, 73, 74, 75
losing weight, 74–5
see also overweight
"wet dreams", 112
whips, bondage, 144
whiteheads, 37, 39
wigs, 44
wine, 19, 77
woman astride position, intercourse, 175, 180
work:
getting out of a rut, 16–17
and impotence, 150
time management, 30
workaholism, 12, 28–31
working hours, 17, 31
wounds, 39
wrinkles, 37

X
X position, intercourse, 181

Y
Y-fronts, 148
yohimbine, 152

Z
zinc, 21, 80, 133
zits, 39
ZZ Top beards, 48

Acknowledgements

Octopus Publishing Group Ltd 55, 104–105, 124–125, 128, 132, 136–137, 139 159, 170–171, 172–173, 174–175, 176–177, 178–179, 180–181, 182–183,/Andreas Einseidel 18–19,/Steve Gorton 32–33, 36–37,/Colin Gotts 6, 9, 84–85, 86–87, 90–91, 98–99, 100–101, 116–117, 121, 122–123, 142–143, 145, 160–161, 168–169,/Paul Grater 21,/Ruth Jenkinson 40–41, 45–51, 89, 134–135,/James Merrell 152–153,/Roger Phillips 70–71, 78–79,/Richard Truscott 50,/Halli Verrinder 38, 53; Rodale Images/J P Hamel 24, 82–83,/Mitch Mandel 10–11, 15, 42–43, 56,/Kurt Wilson 1, 2–3, 4–5, 30–31, 34–35, 92–93, 108–109, 148–149.

Bibliography

Dr Sarah Brewer, *The Complete Book of Men's Health* (Thorsons, London, 1995).
Dr Steve Carroll, *The Which? Guide to Men's Health* (Which? Limited, London, 1999).
Dr David Delvin, *A to Z of Health & Sex* (Ebury Press, London, 1990).
Jack Forem, et al.,*The Complete Book of Men's Health* (Mitchell Beazley, London, 1999).
John Gray, *Men Are From Mars, Women Are From Venus* (Thorsons, London, 1992).
Anne Hooper, *Anne Hooper's Ultimate Sex Guide* (Dorling Kindersley, London, 1992).
Roy Lacey, *The Organic Greenhouse & Conservatory* (David & Charles, London, 1992).
Dr Amanda Roberts, *Reader's Digest Guide to Love & Sex* (The Reader's Digest Association Limited, London, 1998).
Anne Szarewski and John Guillebaud, *Contraception, A User's Handbook* (Oxford University Press, Oxford, 1998).
Hasnain Walji, *Vitamin Guide* (Element Books Limited, Shaftesbury, Dorset, 1992).